PROGRESSIVE CALISTHENICS

The 20-Minute Dream Body with Bodyweight Exercises

By John Powers

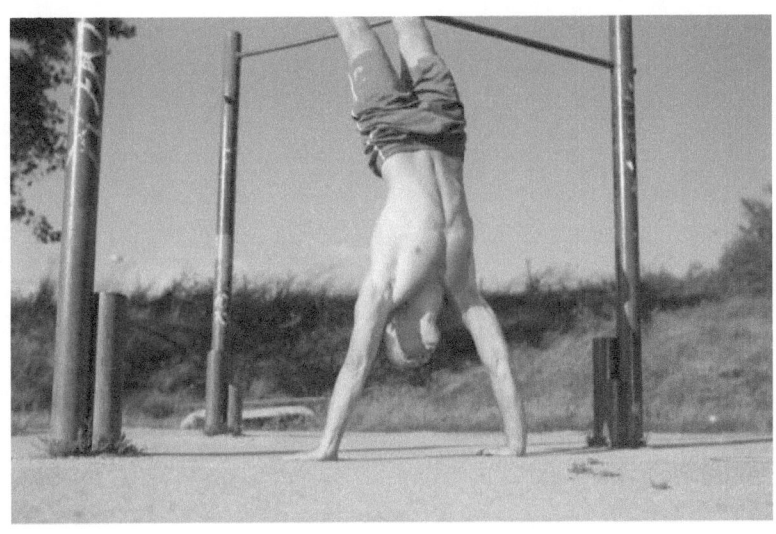

"The individual who says it is not possible should move out of the way of those doing it!"
- Tricia Cunningham

TABLE OF CONTENTS

INTRODUCTION

A great looking body, plenty of strength and agility, and a positive mental outlook are the dream for most people. **For those willing to put in 20 to 30 minutes a day at least 3 days a week performing a variety of calisthenics and bodyweight exercises, the dream can easily become a reality!**

Calisthenics (*Cals*) and ***Bodyweight training*** (*BWT*) have been around since the dawn of time – there were no gyms or fancy exercise equipment! Everyone has seen the movies with Roman gladiators, Greek warriors, and Nordic fighting men, and their physiques are all impressive! These images may come to us today from Hollywood, but the reality is also presented in countless museums across the globe in the shape of statues and paintings of real men and women.

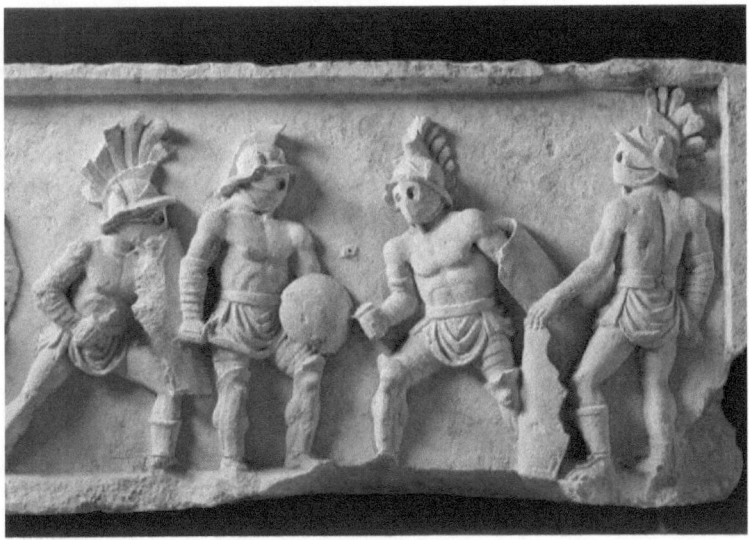

1

There are also plenty of ***modern-day examples*** of excellent levels of fitness achieved primarily through calisthenics and bodyweight training:

- *Gymnasts*
- *Figure skaters*
- *Acrobats*
- *Martial arts experts*

The human body is an amazing machine, and it takes proper nutrition and maintenance in the form of functional movements to keep it functioning at an optimal level. Unfortunately, the availability of handy pre-prepared foods and labor-saving devices have caused people to lose sight of the best ways to keep healthy, and these habits are hard to break.

With just a little practice and determination, it is possible to reverse the effects of improper diet and inadequate activity at virtually any age and **develop a strong, healthy, fit body that looks good and leaves you feeling great**.

In this book, you will be presented with an overview of how the body functions and the benefits calisthenics and bodyweight training provide. ***You will learn about***:

- The differences between Cals and BWT and other types of workouts
- How the body creates and burns energy
- Proper nutrition to fuel the body
- The impact the mind has on the effectiveness of exercise
- How to perform a wide variety of Cals and BWT exercises
- Basic workout routines and how to amp them up

In other words, **you will receive the information and motivation you need to begin a Cals and BWT program and create the body and mental outlook you have only hoped for in the past**. And this is all possible without expensive equipment, gym memberships, or countless hours of exertion.

Happy exercising!

CHAPTER 1

Physical Fitness Throughout History

"It's easier to stay in shape if you never
let yourself get out of shape in the first place."
- Bill Loguidice

There is nothing new about wanting a strong, fit body. Many types of exercise programs and a tremendous number of exercise gadgets and machines have come and gone, but the original form of athletic training, calisthenics and bodyweight activities, are still going strong. **Countless people have developed excellent physiques and unsurpassed stamina through regular bodyweight training, and it doesn't cost a thing!**

ANCIENT TO MODERN TIMES

Physical fitness has been prized since the beginning of time. At first, it was the means by which people were able to provide food and shelter necessary for their survival. Strength and stamina were required for hunting and gathering food, and the nomadic way of life meant that groups were constantly on the move.

Even after the rise of agrarian societies, the rigors of daily life necessitated strength and endurance for plowing fields, harvesting crops, and hauling and storing all types of wares.

As more people became engaged in less strenuous occupations, general fitness levels began to decline. This pattern has existed among the people of the world for over 7,000 years.

Philosophy and religion combined with gymnastics and other forms of physical training in ancient China and India as the correlation between a healthy body and healthy mind was realized. Physical ailments and diseases were found to result from inactivity, and this led to the creation of Kung Fu gymnastics and yoga. The famous Chinese philosopher, educator, and politician *Confucius* is credited with saying that exercise is good for the overall person. Shaolin Monks were highly trained through rigorous calisthenics to be able to defend their monasteries and are considered to be among the most deadly combatants in history.

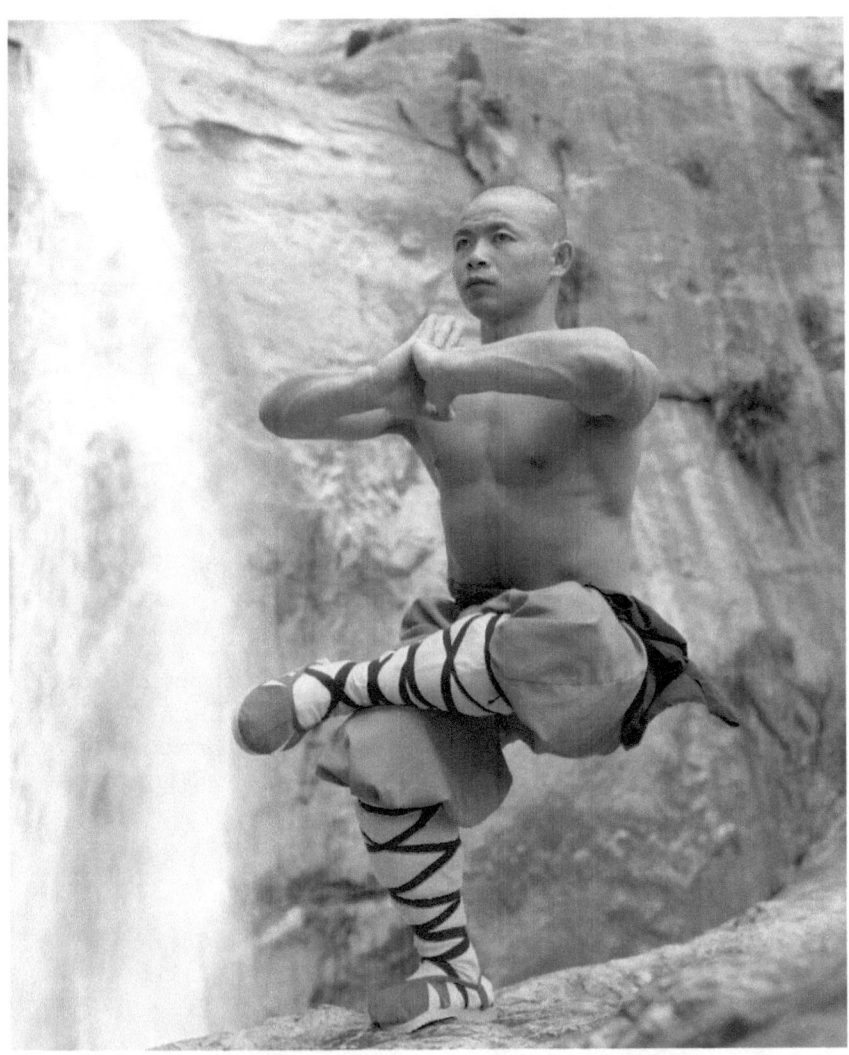

Ancient records and artifacts point to the regular participation of both men and women in athletic pursuits. Pictures found on Egyptian artifacts depict acrobatic activities, and the beauty of the human form was admired by ancient Greeks who believed that a healthy body was necessary for intellectual growth. Men of all ages took advantage of gymnasiums and participated in a variety of contests such as ball games, tug-of-war, and throwing the discus or javelin. This, of course, led to the *Olympic Games* that began in 776 BC and even the *Heraean Games* for women sometime in the sixth century BC.

In numerous cultures, such as the Persian, Spartan, and Roman, strength and fitness were seen as the basic elements necessary for military might.

Anyone who has seen movies such as *300, Troy, Pompeii*, or *Hercules* can appreciate the beautiful musculature and amazing power of the main characters. From a young age, boys were trained for eventual military service, and women were also encouraged to engage in fitness training to ensure the birth of strong, healthy babies.

Interestingly enough, it is also a fact that many of these civilizations declined as the citizens relaxed and enjoyed the wealth and leisure that conquest brought. As physical fitness diminished, early groups were then more easily overthrown by stronger, more able-bodied aggressors.

Moving ahead 1,000 years, the value of good physical conditioning was also recognized by leaders in many different countries. In Europe during the Renaissance (1400-1600), the interest in the culture of the ancient Greeks and Romans sparked an increase in the interest in the human body. Da Vinci's anatomical drawings were the first to clearly identify muscles and explain how the body moves. In the field of medicine and also in relation to the mind-body connection of a well-rounded education, fitness and the proper functioning of the body became important topics of study.

Just a few hundred years later as nations began to develop independently, the importance of a fit citizenry led to the founding of physical education programs and a broad following for gymnastics. England, Germany, Denmark, and Sweden were among the leaders of the creation of fitness programs and clubs designed to improve and maintain the health and physical well-being of all citizens.

EXERCISE IN AMERICA

Early American leaders such as *Benjamin Franklin* and *Thomas Jefferson* also recommended physical activity for the health and well-being of the citizenry. At the beginning of the twentieth century, President *Theodore Roosevelt* used his position as leader of the country to encourage people to participate in a wide variety of athletic activities since that was how he had overcome severe childhood asthma.

Although Americans had begun to participate fairly regularly in sports activities in the post- Civil War years, many people were not really very active. As a result of a more sedentary lifestyle, especially in urban areas, and no organized physical education programs in public schools, it was discovered that the nation as a whole did not meet basic fitness standards. **One out of every 3 men drafted for military service in WWI was found to be unfit** for combat, and almost half of the draftees for WWII were rejected or placed in non-combat posts.

The rise in research involving the minimum muscular fitness of children led by the experts *Drs. Kraus* and *Hirschland,* led to the findings that **almost 60 percent of American children could not pass all of a series of tests** for determining physical fitness compared to only 9 percent of European children where physical education was taught in school. This led to the creation of the *President's Council on Youth Fitness* under President Eisenhower but was later changed to the President's Council on Physical Fitness under President Kennedy who actually wrote an article for *Sports Illustrated* entitled "The Soft American."

The current statistics regarding childhood obesity and physical fitness are alarming. According to government figures, only **30 percent of children are active every day** and almost **17 percent are considered obese**. It is sadly not surprising when only 6 US states require physical education in all grades from kindergarten through 12th in public schools. That inclination toward obesity carries on into adulthood and leads to a wide variety of preventable diseases and conditions.

America Is Fatter Than Ever

Obesity prevalence among adults and youths in the U.S.*

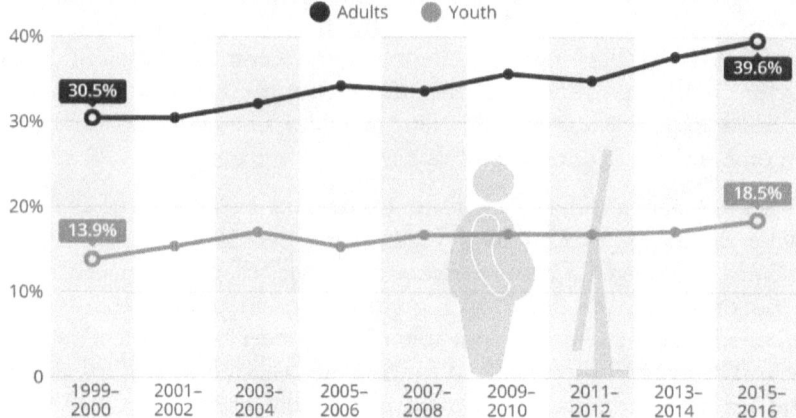

* Adults aged 20 and over and youth aged 2-19 years.
@StatistaCharts   Source: Centers For Disease Control And Prevention

statista

FITNESS AROUND THE WORLD

THE WEIGHT OF THE WORLD

% of population considered overweight or obese

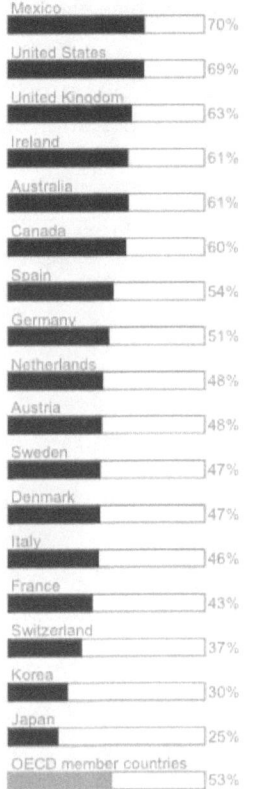

Mexico — 70%
United States — 69%
United Kingdom — 63%
Ireland — 61%
Australia — 61%
Canada — 60%
Spain — 54%
Germany — 51%
Netherlands — 48%
Austria — 48%
Sweden — 47%
Denmark — 47%
Italy — 46%
France — 43%
Switzerland — 37%
Korea — 30%
Japan — 25%
OECD member countries — 53%

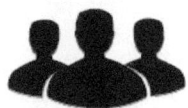

One in three adults in the world (1.46 billion) were overweight or obese in 2008, up by 23% since 1980.

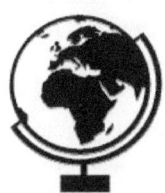

In the developing world, the number of overweight or obese adults more than tripled from 250 million in 1980 to 904 million in 2008.

Across the globe, consumption of sugar and sweeteners rose 20% per person between 1961 and 2009.

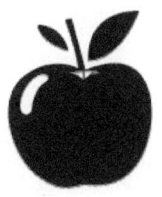

The world's least-developed countries have average diets that fall short of the recommended amounts of fruit, vegetables, dairy and other protein-rich foods such as fish and meat.

Source: OECD, 2010 or most recent data available

Sources: OECD Factbook 2012, United Nations Food and Agriculture Organization, Overseas Development Institute Report: Future Diets

The lack of a healthy diet and inadequate exercise is a problem around the globe. Unfortunately, these two factors play a large role in the development of non-communicable diseases, such as cardiovascular issues, hypertension, cancer, and diabetes, which affect a large percentage of the world's population in both developing and developed countries. Increased urbanization, easy transportation, and an abundance of labor-saving devices in the home have reduced the amount of physical activity for most people. There is also much more focus on sedentary pastimes such as watching TV or playing with computers.

Along with better diet choices, a **daily minimum of 30 minutes of exercise is recommended**. The *World Health Organization* has implemented many programs to promote healthy choices around the world since basic calisthenics and bodyweight exercises have been proven to be quite effective for weight loss and weight management. Simple, functional exercises that are fun to do can go a long way in improving overall health and wellness, increasing emotional well-being and easing the burden on the health system.

A NEW BEGINNING

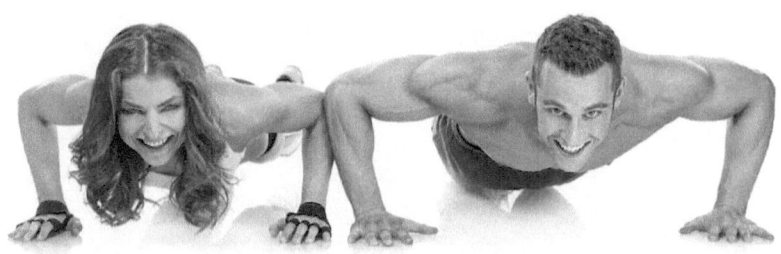

In spite of the abundance of well-advertised exercise programs and fitness equipment, there has been a general decline in the fitness level of many modern people. More and more individuals, though, are beginning to recognize the importance of physical fitness for their health and emotional well-being. That is part of the beauty of calisthenics and bodyweight programs because there is no cost involved and no need for any special equipment. Just like with the hunters, gatherers, and warriors of ancient times, **it is possible to achieve a high level of fitness simply in as little as 20 to 30 minutes a day**!

An easy-to-follow exercise program, tips for motivation, and an improved diet are the goals of this book. Even if you think there isn't enough time in your day, you will discover that many of these exercises can be done while waiting in traffic, sitting at work, watching TV, or even doing the dishes. Once you begin to feel a difference in your attitude as well as the fit of your clothes, you will be happy to carve out a bit more time every day to achieve results that you never thought were possible without a gym membership or expensive equipment. **You are certainly worth the effort, and you will have the rest of your life to enjoy the results!**

CHAPTER 2

What Are Calisthenics (Cals) And Bodyweight Training (BWT)

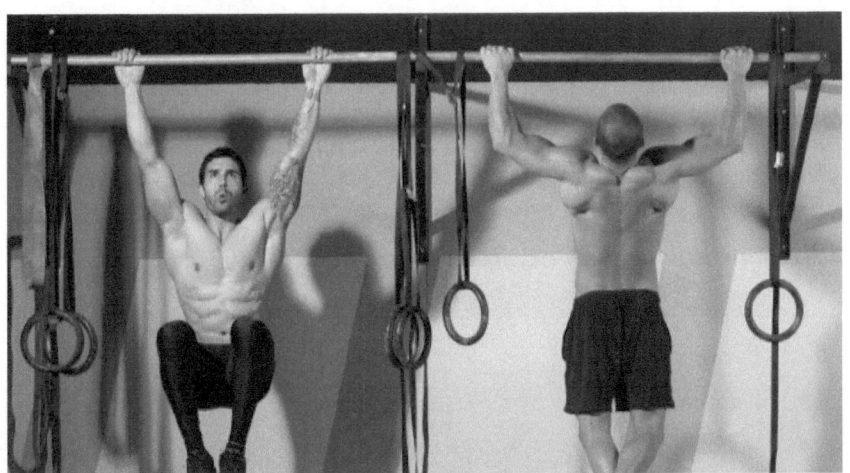

When asked this question, many people may think of the exercises they used to do in gym class. Jumping jacks, push-ups, sit-ups, and squats were the bane of the school child's day! While those activities are part of the overall picture of calisthenics and bodyweight training, there is so much more! And now, it can even be fun!

CALS AND BWT DEFINED

Calisthenics, from the Greek '*kalos*' for **beautiful** and '*sthenos*' for **strength**, refers to exercises that incorporate simple, natural body movements using only the weight of your body as resistance to increase strength, flexibility, mobility, agility, and endurance. It is a matter of learning to control your body for optimal results, but the basics are easy for anyone, male or female, young or old. **Bodyweight training** is simply another name for the calisthenics activities because of the fact that only the weight of your body is used to perform the exercises.

Although there are technically only a few basic exercises, there are countless variations of them to keep things interesting. The alternatives come from modifications that increase the difficulty of the moves or target more slightly different muscles. **Injury is uncommon** since you are controlling your own movements and don't have any weights or machines to get in the way or cause a strain.

The beauty of calisthenics is that it depends completely on your own body weight and involves functional motions – full range movements that are natural for all the activities you perform daily. Along with improved general fitness, adding calisthenics to your daily routine will help you lose weight and inches, gain lean muscle mass and tone, and improve your cardiovascular health with greater endurance.

Movements involved in calisthenics include:

- Accelerating and decelerating
- Bending
- Jumping
- Kicking
- Pulling and pushing
- Squatting
- Swinging
- Twisting

When you look at the range of calisthenics movements, you will discover that *aerobics, gymnastics, Pilates, running, yoga, martial arts,* and *walking* are all actually considered **calisthenics activities**. The preparation for all of these activities begins with the very basic movements that are included in the playlist for calisthenics. By mastering the basics, creating modifications, and perfecting control of your body, you are automatically preparing for better performance in any sport or activity.

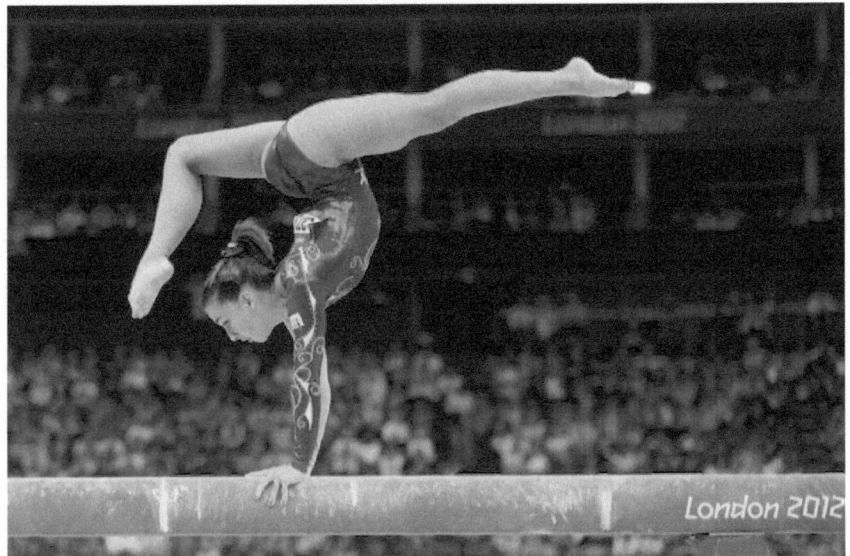

London 2012

Just by thinking of these disciplines, you can get the picture of how the movements can be modified for greater difficulty. A simple bridge becomes a back walkover to a gymnast and controlled jumping jacks can be transferred to karate chops and kicks. Pilates and Yoga moves are generally slower and more controlled than other forms of calisthenics and combine with mental concentration for a meditative experience. While Yoga focuses on balance, posture and stretches, Pilates concentrates more on the core and powerhouse muscles of the hips and buttocks. Aerobics classes are a dynamic form of calisthenics usually set to music and even dance – from ballet to modern and just look at break dancers! – and depend on the coordinated functioning of the body in a wide range of motions. The same comparisons can be made with figure skaters and acrobats such as *Cirque du Soleil* performers.

THE COMBINATION OF ISOMETRICS AND PLYOMETRICS

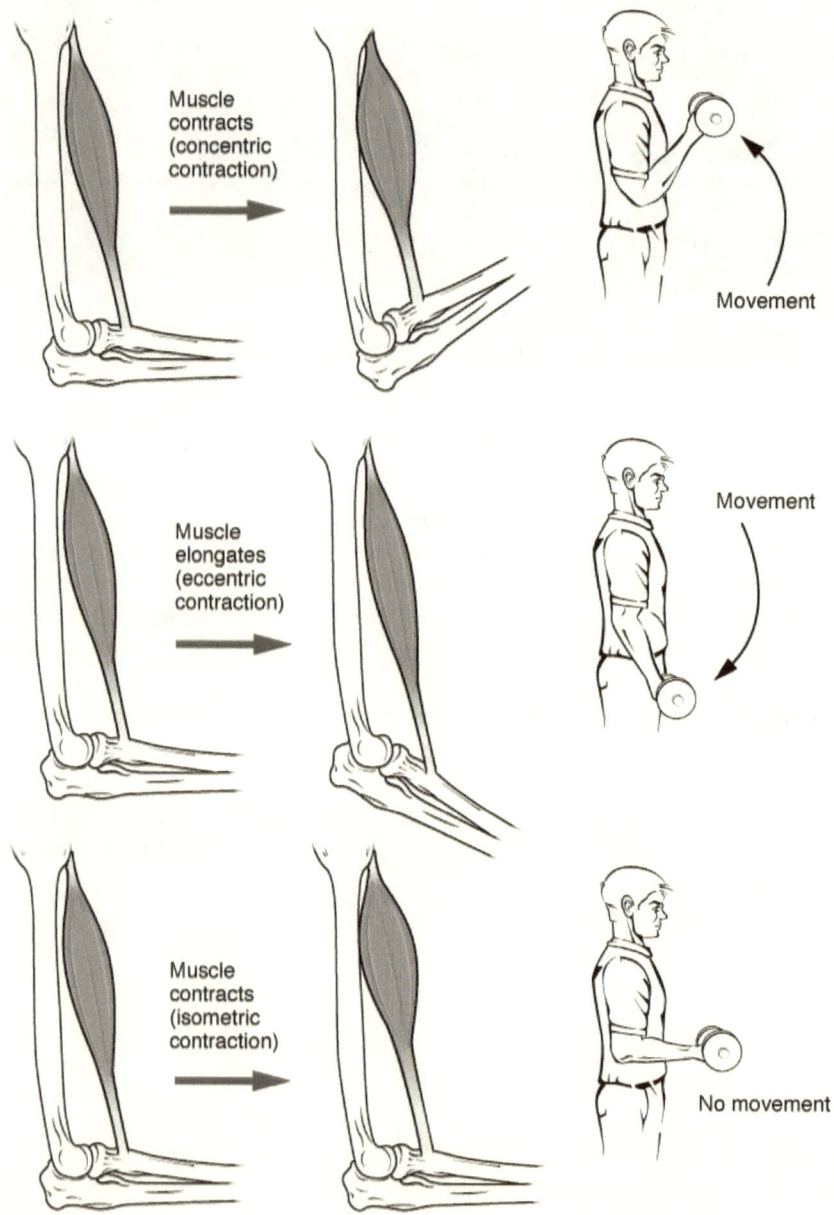

Muscle contracts (concentric contraction)

Movement

Muscle elongates (eccentric contraction)

Movement

Muscle contracts (isometric contraction)

No movement

In addition to simply moving – using your muscles and increasing heart rate – **calisthenics and bodyweight exercises include the principles of isometrics and plyometrics**. These activities help maximize the effectiveness of Cals and BWT workouts and help to increase strength and muscle mass.

Isometric exercise sounds contradictory – a workout without moving. What this really means is that you hold a position for 10 to 20 or even up to 60 seconds, which contracts certain muscles. This contraction is the actual 'work.' Isometrics are low impact and are great for beginners or people rehabbing from injury because you can only work the muscle as far as your strength and condition allow. There is no equipment required, and these exercises can be done anywhere.

A variety of **motions** are **involved in performing isometric exercises**:

- Pushing against an immovable object such as a wall

- Holding up an object (weight, medicine ball) or even just an arm or leg and not letting it lower

- Holding a position (either pushing, pulling, or holding a load) as long as possible – 20 to 60 seconds (good for the development of muscle mass)

- Applying maximum tension to an immovable object for up to 6 seconds (Creating the contraction quickly improves strength, muscle mass, and torque but can lead to a strain and is usually done by athletes for increased speed and explosiveness.)

- Combining static/dynamic positions such as a runner pushing off the block or holding the down-position of a push-up and quickly extending the arms (good for explosive strength and speed – great for martial arts)

Plyometric exercises, on the other hand, increase muscular power, speed, and explosiveness. Since this involves the quick stretch of muscles followed by a quick shortening, plyometric exercises can cause injuries if the proper preparation is not performed. Specific training with plyometrics is used by professional athletes to improve performance in sports such as football, basketball, tennis, skiing, and boxing or martial arts, which require rapid changes in position, direction, and speed.

Simply stated, *plyometric exercises involve hopping, skipping, and jumping*. A dip before a jump adds significantly to the muscle workout by contracting then releasing the muscle. The benefits of this move are explained as either a *coil reflex* (like compressing then releasing a spring) or a stretch reflex where the body instinctively tries to prevent over-stretching making the contracting movement more forceful in response.

Repetitive plyometric training leads to quicker, stronger muscle contraction and that means better athletic performance. But even relative beginners can take advantage of the concept of plyometrics in basic exercises to add an element of difficulty to their workout.

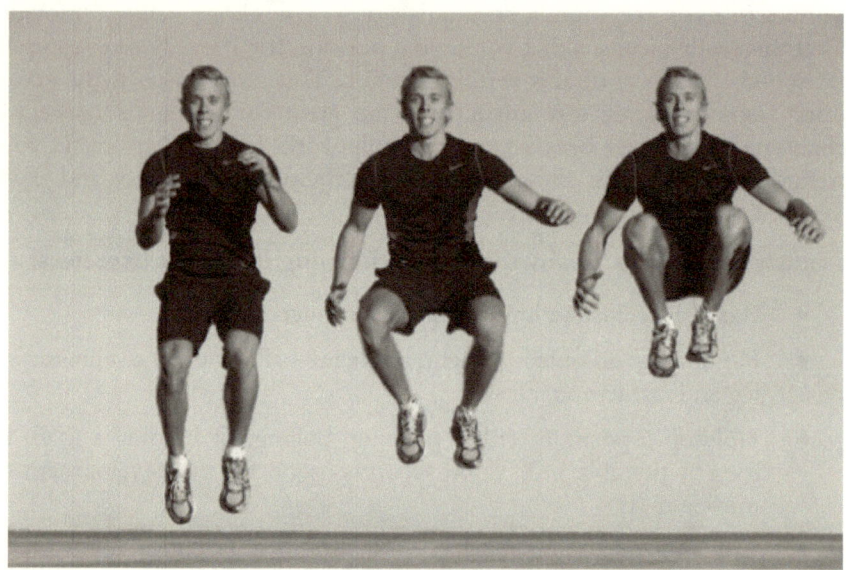

ADVANTAGES AND BENEFITS OF CALS AND BWT

Over the years, most people turned away from calisthenics because they were more impressed with machines, fancy gyms, or special programs. When you get past the hype about the latest 'fad,' you are back to the basics – Cals and bodyweight exercises. In a relatively short period of time and with no investment of money, you can effectively tone and strengthen your body while losing weight and inches since these exercises can turn your body into a fat-burning machine.

Cals and BWT involve both **aerobic and anaerobic activities** and that is where **the true fat burning potential** of these workouts lies. The functional nature of the movements involved in calisthenics and bodyweight exercises provide synergistic benefits to the muscles and CNS (*Central Nervous System*).

Among the many *advantages of calisthenics and bodyweight exercises* are:

- Completely free, require no equipment and can be done anytime, anywhere
- Appropriate for people of all ages and abilities
- Increase overall agility, balance, coordination, energy, stamina, and strength
- Neural adaptation occurs quickly allowing for a faster increase in strength
- Promote complete body fitness – physical and mental (Exercise is a great mood lifter!)
- Help burn fat and build lean muscle mass
- Strengthen muscles that support joints, allowing you to be more stable and avoid injury
- Also strengthen skeletal and cardiac muscles
- Offer relief from a variety of body aches and pains
- Provide a completely balanced workout for the entire body
- Improve the immune response of the body to help prevent a number of diseases
- Reduce the risk of developing a hernia due to excessive weight

DISADVANTAGES OF CALS AND BWT

Just to be fair, let's look at what *some* people consider to be disadvantages of this type of exercise. It is *claimed* that you will not increase muscle mass quickly with Cals and BWT since these exercises don't provide many opportunities for focusing on specific muscles. It is also *believed* (mistakenly) that boredom can set in with the apparently limited number of exercises you can do and that the inability to add weight for more resistance limits your ultimate success.

So, if you really want to add muscle and get big, especially quickly, some '*experts*' say you should stick with weights and machines. But **if you are more interested in strong, well-defined muscles, a low BMI (*Body Mass Index*), great abs, and an overall toned and fit body, then keep reading!**

CALISTHENICS AND BODYWEIGHT TRAINING DO IT ALL

Let's take another look at the concept of **synergy** – the linking together of movements and exercises to combine the benefits to a wider range of muscles. While this can be accomplished to a limited degree with machines and weights by taking advantage of the synergy between the contraction (positive) and stretching (negative) aspects of the exercise, the nature of Cals and BWT provide plenty of interaction between different muscle groups at all times.

The body is an amazing machine that rivals anything the gym has to offer. It is capable of complex motions in what are called the '**6 Degrees of Freedom**,' a concept that is applied to the movement of the human body, an airplane or rocket, and a robot in and through three-dimensions:

- Moving forward and backward - *surging*

- Moving up and down - *heaving*

- Moving side to side - *swaying*

- Rotating around the up and down axis (turning left and right) – *yawing*

- Tilting forward and backward – *pitching*

- Tilting side to side – *rolling*

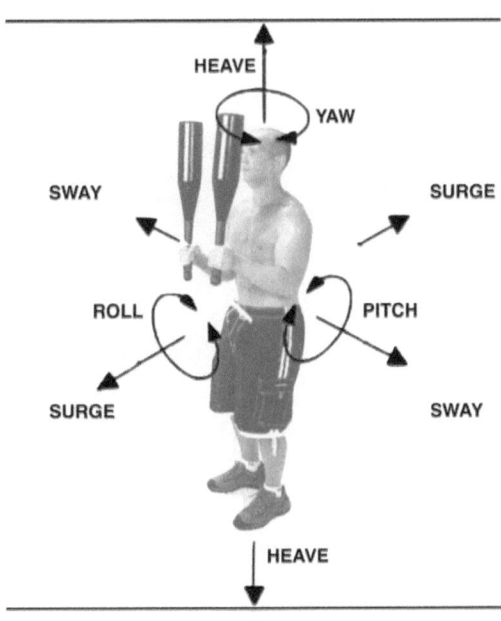

It is through these movements that **you can ensure a full range of mobility and utilize the most muscles**. This contributes to improved balance and overall strength, both of which are important for good physical fitness and to avoid injury. Machines and weights isolate muscles and can lead to imbalance as well as inefficiency when confronted with a need for speed since the muscles are held in a static position.

Machines provide support for the body while working isolated muscles. In comparison, bodyweight exercises involve not only the leg muscles, for example, but also engage the core muscles – the abs, obliques, and hip flexors. Not only are muscles worked, their supporting tendons and ligaments are activated and better overall fitness is achieved. With constant minute adaptations to conditions during Cals and BWT, the body becomes better able to handle everyday activities or adjust to any unexpected situation such as slipping on the ice or even walking over uneven terrain.

THE CORRELATION BETWEEN STRENGTH AND MUSCLE MASS

When choosing a workout routine, the first question you need to consider is **whether you are interested in increasing strength and overall fitness or developing massive muscles**. Calisthenics and bodyweight exercises can build muscle throughout the entire body but not necessarily the type you see in pictures of body builders and *Mr. Universe* contestants. **Cals and BWT develop lean muscle mass that has more power than the muscles of super-huge guys and gals.**

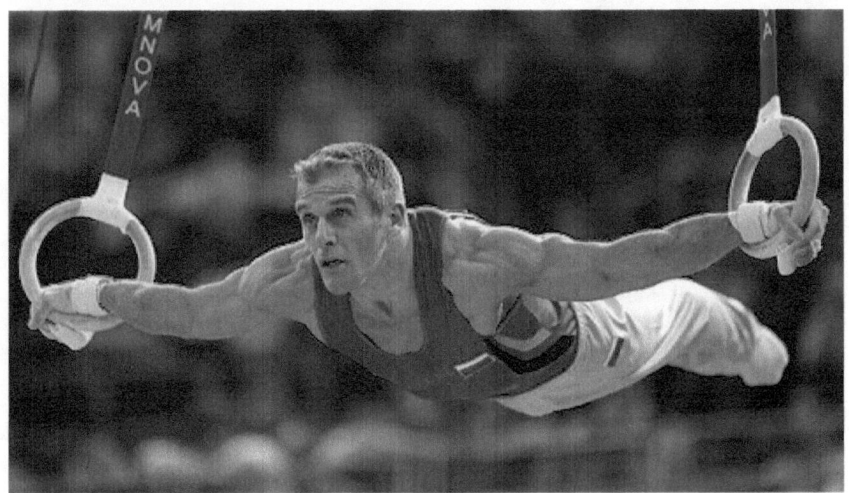

Compare the body of a gymnast to that of a body builder. The gymnast is able to hold his or her bodyweight through a wide variety of disciplines involving the entire body over an extended period of time. This is what is known as *deceptive strength* – you would not expect the body to be able to perform these feats. The iron cross on the rings or one-handed handstands, not to mention consecutive flips across the mat or flying on the pommel horse or uneven bars are standard skills all gymnasts have mastered with the functional exercises of Cals and BWT.

BODYBUILDING

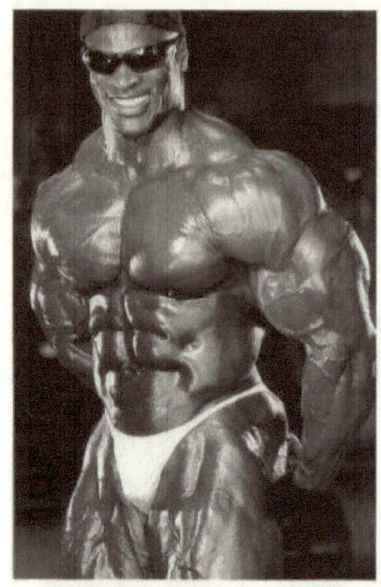

STREET WORKOUT

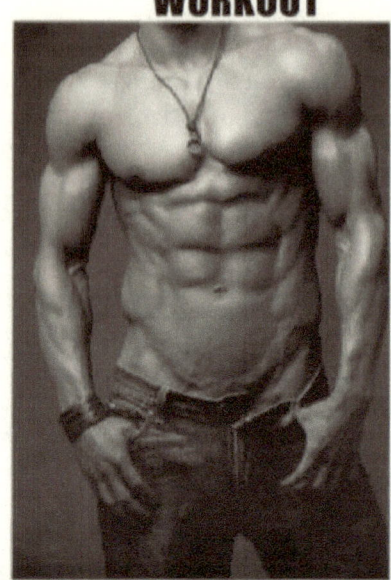

LEARN THE DIFFERENCE !

Most sports and activities require a combination of *nervous system* and *muscular system* training. Calisthenics and bodyweight exercises provide both due to the ability to tailor each exercise to your particular goals.

For relatively inexperienced people, the focus should be on nervous system training – getting the body used to the demands for specific routines and exercises. This is important because training properly is the key to ultimate success, and it is in these early stages that many bad habits can be formed.

In nervous system training, the cells are taught to communicate more efficiently so that the desired movements are easier and automatic. This occurs typically with **low reps (1-5) but frequent sets** during which the exercises are performed as perfectly as possible as many times as you can. The end result is skill development as the nervous system reconfigures itself for optimum performance.

Muscular system training is different because it **focuses on the growth of muscle cells through the progressive increase of chemical energy**. By pushing the muscles to their limits with **multiple reps (6-15) and only one or a few sets**, this energy is constantly depleted, and the result is muscle growth during rest periods. You are actually forcing your muscles to adapt to these increased demands by growing in size and strength. Therefore you should pick a challenging exercise and push yourself as hard as you can. Note that adequate rest periods are needed for the muscular system to recover.

If you are looking for a secret to the success of calisthenics and bodyweight training, it can be summed up in one word – **control**. The ability to train and control your muscles to make them do what you want is the goal of Cals and BWT, and that is where a mature, well-planned program is so vastly different from what we all remember of grammar school phys. ed. class. Your goals and individual creativity determine the fun and success you have with a program of calisthenics and bodyweight training.

CHAPTER 3

How The Body Adapts To Exercise

The great news is that any regular **calisthenics (Cals) or bodyweight training (BWT) program can improve your fitness with visible results in four to eight weeks**. The bad news is that you must maintain a certain percentage of that level of activity to prevent losing what you have worked so hard to gain. That's just the way it is. The even better news, though, is that a basic program of Cals and BWT is something that you can do easily anywhere, anytime and for the rest of your life.

THE BODY IS AN INTEGRATED WHOLE

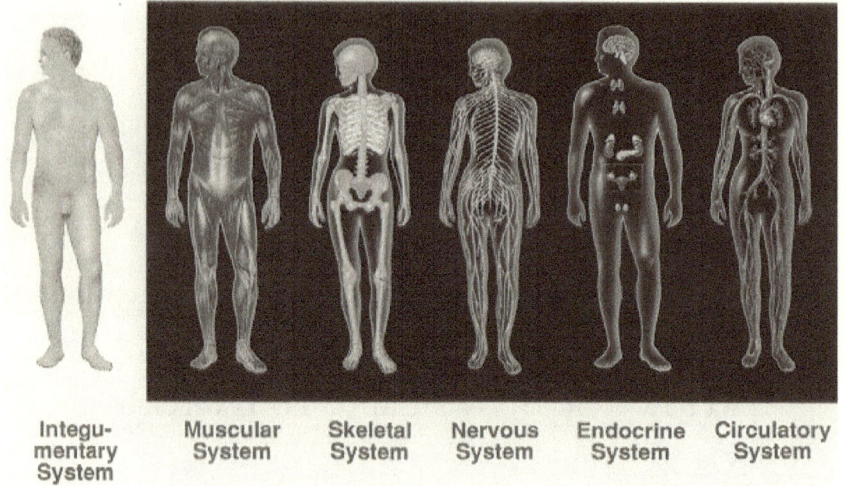

| Integu-mentary System | Muscular System | Skeletal System | Nervous System | Endocrine System | Circulatory System |

Everything you do – even the way you think – has some effect on another system or part of the body. Everything works together to provide for the most efficient functioning possible and that functioning can be fine-tuned with a healthy diet and regular exercise. The result is better overall health and fitness.

Muscle activity is just one factor that comes into play during calisthenics and bodyweight exercise. Your heart rate and breathing rate change, nerves fire faster, and blood flows quicker. Hormones are released, fat stores are broken down for energy, and your metabolism responds to greater demands. You get a little sweaty and maybe feel a bit sore, but your mood is improved, and you actually look forward to doing it all over.

Every individual is just that – a unique person with his or her own genetics and physical capabilities that will determine the actual results of diet and exercise. In spite of the differences, there are many different physiological factors that work together within each person to shape the body and run its many systems. While the most obvious changes occur to the cardiovascular system and the muscles, there are also considerable benefits to the endocrine, immune, and metabolic systems as well.

MUSCLES MAKE YOU MOVE

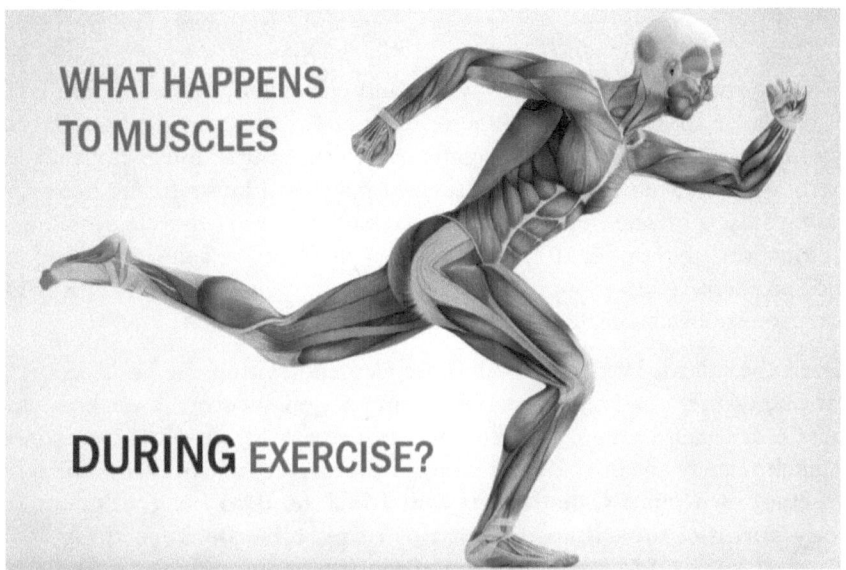

The human body contains over 600 muscles, and getting them to work together in groups happens naturally up to a point. All healthy individuals manage to walk and move in ways that enable them to provide food and self-care. **The difference between the 'average' person and an athlete is the degree to which the muscles are trained for specific purposes**.

The mechanics of movement involve the contraction of one muscle and the relaxation of another, called the *antagonist*. With exercise, the muscles work in unison, and the more repetitions that are performed, the more natural the actions become. The muscle fibers grow and can actually increase in number when enough resistance is encountered over a period of time.

Even muscles that we cannot consciously control benefit from exercise. The striated muscles of the skeletal system (anything that is attached to a bone) come under voluntary control, but the smooth or visceral muscles of the organs like the digestive system as well as the cardiac muscle – the heart – function without conscious control for as long as the body is alive. They depend on the fresh oxygen and nutrients supplied by good blood flow to keep working at maximum efficiency.

It is not just the muscles that control movement, however. Tendons that connect muscles to bones and ligaments, which connect one bone to another, help support the body, protect the joints, and allow for movement by anchoring the muscles to withstand the contractions that cause bending, sliding rotation, and all the other motions involved in moving the body.

Another component of our bodies that has an effect on our overall comfort, fitness, and ability to move is the *myofascia*. This is a connective web of tissue that creates the organ cavities and membranes and provides a covering for the muscles and bones. The myofascia of each individual is different and responds to the physical and emotional stresses of the body. In times of extreme stress, illness, or trauma, the sympathetic nervous system causes the myofascia to contract. If this contraction is not relieved, the body will experience musculoskeletal pains and knots to the point that the myofascia of one muscle attaches to that of another muscle, resulting in a reduction of motion, decreased energy, difficulty relaxing and sleeping, and problems with concentration at the very least, or an orthopedic compromise or chronic pain if the problem persists.

Given the interdependence of all these elements within the body, injury to any one of them can have a significant impact on another. A weakness in a muscle can cause strain to the connective tissue or an injured tendon or ligament can result in the weakening of the muscle or an alteration to the structure of a joint. **Calisthenics and BWT tend to be gentler on the body and its joints than other types of exercise because there is no external force added to the range of motion of the muscles**.

HOW THE MUSCLES ARE CONTROLLED

All muscle activity, whether voluntary or involuntary, is controlled by the messages sent to and from the brain through your nervous system, comprised of the spinal cord and brain – the *Central Nervous System* (CNS) – and all the other nerve fibers that branch out from the CNS to the rest of your body – the *Peripheral Nervous System* (PNS).

The PNS is further broken down into the *Somatic Nervous System* (SNS), which is responsible for virtually all voluntary muscle movements (what you want the muscle to do) and the *Autonomic Nervous System* (ANS), which is responsible for all involuntary muscle function such as the heartbeat, breathing, and digestion.

In another breakdown, the ANS is divided into the *sympathetic system*, which is commonly known by the term 'fight or flight,' and the *parasympathetic system*, which governs normal body function, rest, and the conservation of physical resources.

In the simplest terms, **exercising puts the body in a state of stress that activates the sympathetic nervous system.**

The most common ***attributes of this 'fight or flight' response include:***

- Increase in heart and respiratory rate
- Constriction of many blood vessels not involved in movement
- Dilation of blood vessels in the muscles (to provide more oxygen and nutrients)
- Release of glucose and fat into the bloodstream for energy
- Decrease in the digestive process
- Dilation of pupils and loss of peripheral vision (to increase focus)
- Reduction in the ability to hear (to avoid distraction)

Fight-or-Flight Response

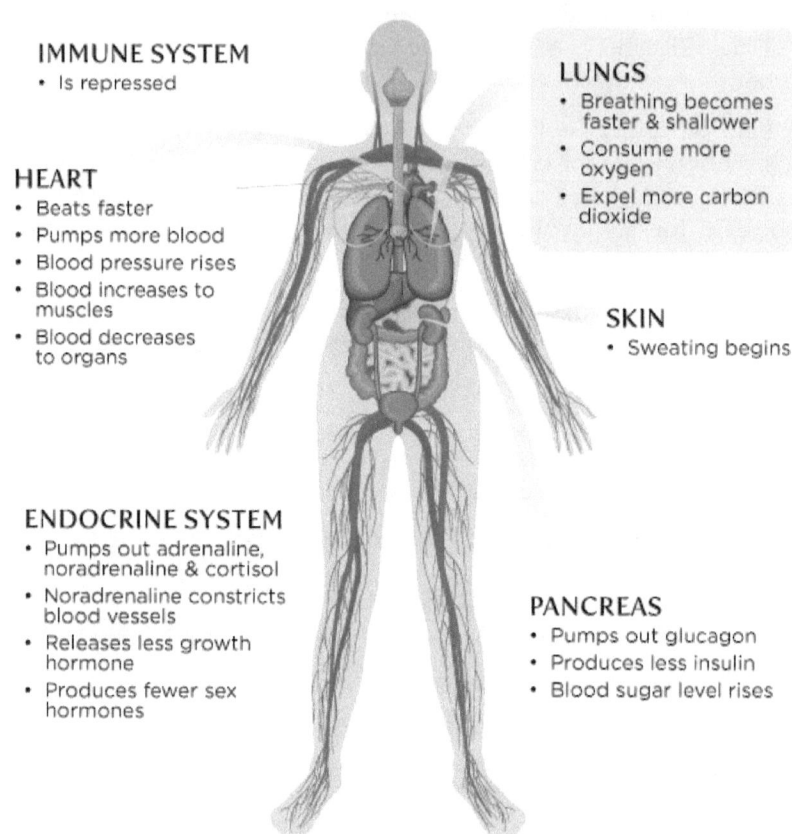

IMMUNE SYSTEM
- Is repressed

LUNGS
- Breathing becomes faster & shallower
- Consume more oxygen
- Expel more carbon dioxide

HEART
- Beats faster
- Pumps more blood
- Blood pressure rises
- Blood increases to muscles
- Blood decreases to organs

SKIN
- Sweating begins

ENDOCRINE SYSTEM
- Pumps out adrenaline, noradrenaline & cortisol
- Noradrenaline constricts blood vessels
- Releases less growth hormone
- Produces fewer sex hormones

PANCREAS
- Pumps out glucagon
- Produces less insulin
- Blood sugar level rises

When the body is ready for activity and these effects take place, you are primed for **optimal muscle function**. Compare some of these features to how you feel or what you see in professional athletes as they prepare to take the field or start a competition. By performing regular exercise, you are able to lessen the strength of the sympathetic nervous response to the point where you can control it but also increase the activation of the parasympathetic or recovery response afterwards. In other words, a little effort up front leads to more benefits down the line.

For the greatest muscle development, it is important to engage the nervous system. Practicing any movement repeatedly helps to establish a pattern for optimal muscle firing – stimulating contractions and relaxations with stabilizers and neutralizers with the right amount of force, in the right order, at the right times. Motor units are groups of muscle fibers within a muscle that are attached to a motor neuron – the pathway for information from the brain. By adding force, you call more motor units into action, and the repeated demand teaches those motor units to function in combination. This results in increased strength and power.

One tremendous benefit of exercise is the increase in the strength of ligaments and tendons, which in turn leads to greater bone density. As the tendons and ligaments pull against the bone, the stress causes bone density growth and is ideal for preventing breaks, especially among older women.

CARDIOVASCULAR BENEFITS OF EXERCISE

All muscles depend on blood flow to provide fluids, oxygen, and nutrients to the cells as well as the removal of cellular waste products for optimal performance. The heart is a muscle that requires the same care as any other muscle. With increased exercise, it is able to pump more blood due to a faster heart rate and greater stroke volume – the amount of blood pushed out with each beat.

Even at rest, the heart pumps more blood after exercise, but the heart rate and blood pressure will decrease. There is also an increase in blood volume, the blood thins, existing capillaries change to allow more blood to flow through larger openings, and new capillaries are formed to provide more blood to the muscles to perform their increased work. Due to the involvement of the sympathetic nervous system, blood flow to the skeletal muscles and skin increases from merely 20% to nearly 80%, and the increase in blood volume helps with this alteration. Additionally, sections of the heart muscle, specifically in the left ventricle, increase in thickness so that they can produce a more forceful contraction to push a greater volume of blood.

Hormones are responsible for signaling the muscles and circulatory system to make the changes that enhance physical performance. It takes a few minutes for these effects to occur so **warming up and cooling down are both important steps in the exercise process**. A rapid change from inactivity to exertion or suddenly ending exercise can result respectively in breathlessness and strains since there is inadequate blood flow or lightheadedness and cramps due to blood lingering in the working muscles since contractions no longer help pump it back to the heart.

To sum it all up, *exercising improves cardiovascular health, which provides these essential benefits*:

1. Reduction of cardiovascular diseases such as high blood pressure and stroke

2. Reduction of visceral body fat that can lead to obesity, diabetes, and several types of cancer

3. Reduction of the effects of stress such as anxiety, depression, and poor sleep

4. Reduction in the need for visits to the doctor and the expense of medical interventions

5. Improvement in the efficiency of all bodily systems through better circulation

6. Enhancement of physical and mental performance due to greater

endurance and focus

7.   Improved self-esteem, body image, and mental outlook

IT IS NOT AS DIFFICULT AS YOU THINK

These are major changes to the body, and the benefits are extreme, so it must be hard to do, right? **No – it is much simpler than you think**! Even for a total couch potato, it only takes 20 to 30 minutes 3 or 4 days a week to be able to see great results in as little as 4 weeks. And it does not mean crazy moves or a killer pace!

```
Couch potato commercial break workout

Option 1

15 Squats

15 Lunges (each leg)

15 Push Ups


Option 2

15 Squat Jumps

5 Plank Hold

25 Jumping Jacks


Option 3

10 Bench Dips

10 Crunches

5 Pull Ups
```

In Chapters 7 and 8, there will be a complete description of exercises and sample workout programs for every skill level – beginners to experienced athletes. Don't worry about the fancy stuff – the important thing is to make the decision to get healthy and get started!

Mental preparation is a big part of successful training so turn the page and learn more about the mind's connection to the body.

CHAPTER 4

The Mind Is A Powerful Tool

For beginners and even seasoned athletes who sometimes hit plateaus, **the mind is an important tool for determining the success of an exercise program**. After all, if engaging in exercise was loads of fun or promised fantastic results easily, more people would be willing to do it without question!

Since you are reading this book, you probably are looking for a way to get fit and need some encouragement as well as instructions. That's where the mind comes into the equation – convincing yourself to take that first step and get involved – in other words, motivation.

OUR SEDENTARY LIFESTYLE

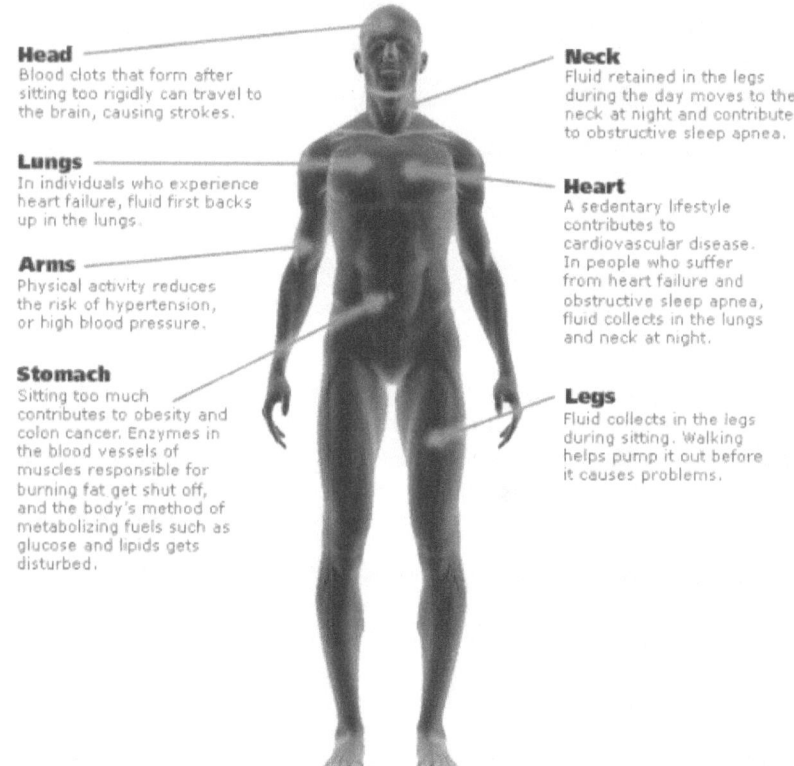

How Sitting Too Long Affects the Body

Head
Blood clots that form after sitting too rigidly can travel to the brain, causing strokes.

Lungs
In individuals who experience heart failure, fluid first backs up in the lungs.

Arms
Physical activity reduces the risk of hypertension, or high blood pressure.

Stomach
Sitting too much contributes to obesity and colon cancer. Enzymes in the blood vessels of muscles responsible for burning fat get shut off, and the body's method of metabolizing fuels such as glucose and lipids gets disturbed.

Neck
Fluid retained in the legs during the day moves to the neck at night and contributes to obstructive sleep apnea.

Heart
A sedentary lifestyle contributes to cardiovascular disease. In people who suffer from heart failure and obstructive sleep apnea, fluid collects in the lungs and neck at night.

Legs
Fluid collects in the legs during sitting. Walking helps pump it out before it causes problems.

One of the primary reasons that exercise is considered work is that we are becoming more and more accustomed to performing less and less physical activity. Not only do most of us have less physically demanding jobs than in years past, we also choose less active leisure pursuits such as going to clubs, watching TV or movies, or playing on the internet or with computer games.

Unlike in some cultures or in 'the old days,' we ride instead of walk, even a few blocks, to the convenience store. We don't even go shopping anymore – we order virtually everything online and wait for it to be delivered!

That is a lot of unused muscle and poorly tuned cardiovascular systems sitting around waiting to get sick and die! Without improving our general fitness level, not to mention dietary habits, we are looking at a very unhealthy future and have begun to see it already with the mounting percentage of obese people with all sorts of preventable illnesses such as diabetes, high blood pressure, and stroke.

Our desire for instant gratification also creates a mental block towards exercise since results take some time. Suzy or John can eat a cupcake or drink a beer and be happy right away, but they have to exercise for a month to see any difference in the way their clothes fit. So, they keep eating those cupcakes and drinking those beers, and in a month, they still need new clothes – just larger sizes!

Now you can see the importance of the proper frame of mind and attitude for making the decision to eat healthy and begin exercising.

GETTING STARTED IS THE HARDEST STEP

Some people feel that they have to jump right in to a rigorous program with extreme goals so that they can get fit. It may be possible, but that approach tends to cause more people to burn out rather quickly, and the program is dropped before anything positive can be achieved.

For the best results, it is recommended that you make small changes over a period of time. In this way, you can come to accept new foods, eating habits, and exercises into your routine with as little fuss as possible. It is a matter of gradually changing the habits you have developed over your lifetime, so you have to give yourself a little leeway in incorporating a switch in your way of doing things.

As you realize that little changes won't hurt you, you can add more new elements to your weekly and daily routines so that they become the automatic fundamentals of your life. Everyone has heard the suggestions before – now it is time to really listen to them and accept them as the lifeline to gaining fitness. You know exactly what they are, too!

- Use stairs instead of elevators – but that does not mean 16 floors!
- Park farther away and walk – or try to get to the corner store on foot!
- Drink more water to curb hunger, especially before meals – it's good for the body, too!
- Eat more fruits and vegetables and cut out fried foods – eat an extra veggie instead of a potato, and leave off the butter, sour cream, and sauces.

If nothing else, be honest with yourself. Do you really like the way you look or feel? There is so much talk about the bad influence of skinny models on women's self-esteem, but that doesn't mean you should give up and let yourself blow up! It's okay if you are not a size 2, but you don't have to become a size 20! Simply, that is Rule Number 1 – **be realistic**! Not all women are going to be top fashion models and not all men will look like Mr. Universe. Those people live their lives to look like that. You live your life for lots of other reasons, and being healthy is the best way to actually just live your life and enjoy the things that you do.

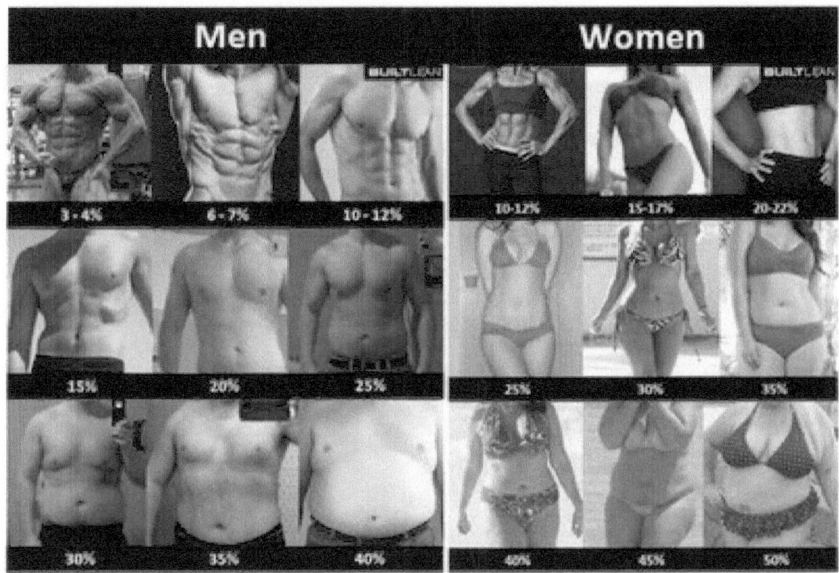

When you make the decision to change, the changes themselves will help keep you on track. With your diet, you will learn what healthy choices taste best so you don't feel as though you are missing out on something. The fact that you look and feel better will become the motivation to continue making healthy choices. Following Rule Number 1 – being realistic – will help you overcome 'guilt' if you indulge once in a while. You can still enjoy a treat but just not one as big or as often.

As you feel better and can sustain activity longer without feeling wiped out, you will enjoy activity more and will make it part of your life. You can still play computer games, but, just like with food, you won't do it as often or as long. You will discover that you have more energy throughout the day and things that always wore you out can now be accomplished much easier. A good workout will encourage you to eat better, and a new positive cycle replaces the old negative one. Once you overcome bad habits involving your diet and exercise choices, you may also find the motivation to tackle other bad habits that may threaten your health such as smoking, drinking, or even work routines that bring about stress. It is even probable that your sex life will improve!

Start small. It is that simple. Look at your everyday life and see when and where you could change something you already do to make it more active. Consider all the time that is wasted in the course of a day and try to plan for more efficiency – even to save 10 minutes here or there so you could take a quick walk or do some stretches. Honestly evaluate the amount of time you spend on the phone, reading emails, watching TV, or simply staring into space. There is undoubtedly enough time every day for a 20-to-30-minute workout. It is a matter of identifying your priorities and putting some things aside.

Now that you are ready to begin, remember that it is always your choice whether or not to continue. You only have to answer to yourself and take only the size steps you want to take – like getting into the water: toe first, then foot, etc. You do not have to jump right in and make major changes all at once.

KEEPING IT GOING

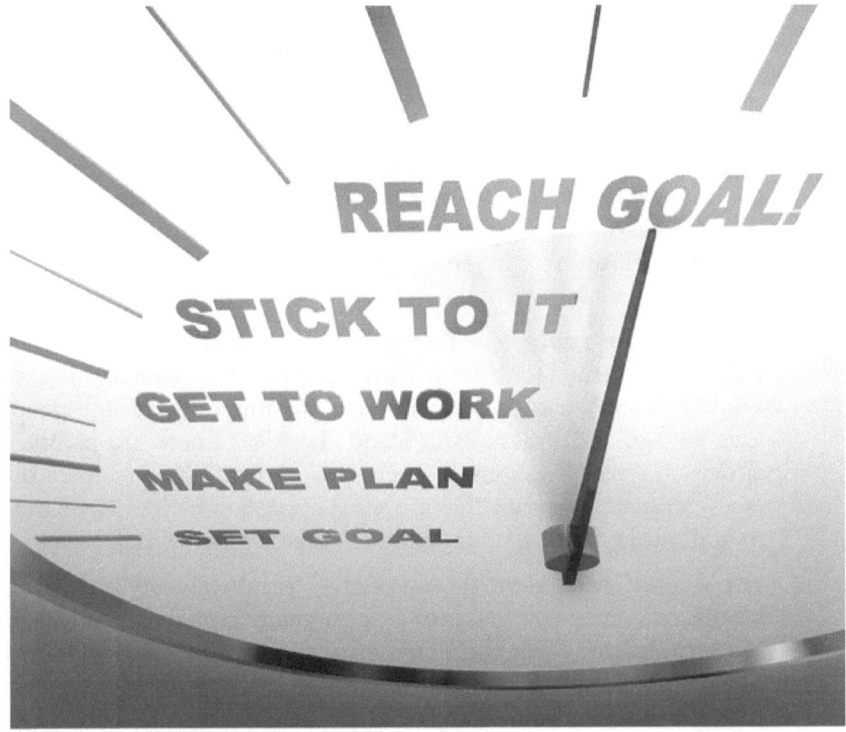

There are countless books about motivation, but the problem is that you have to read them. Not only that, you have to buy into what they are saying and make the changes in your life they recommend. Unfortunately, **there is no magic trick to 'becoming motivated'** so it is up to each individual to find something that works.

Before tackling the mountain of hints for staying motivated, look at some basic mental choices you can make using your own personal values and beliefs.

- *Avoid negative thinking* – Don't look at exercise like a sentence to a work detail! If you go into it hating the whole idea, you will be sure to make it miserable and then tell yourself you were right – it was horrible. Think about having fun doing whatever you choose to do and congratulate yourself as you see yourself succeeding.

- *Think about the results*, not the 'struggle' to get there – Adopt a positive image as you get ready to exercise instead of focusing on how tired or sore you think you will feel. Unlike many other things in life, focus on the destination and not on the steps of the journey, or at least find the fun things on the journey and enjoy them! Almost everything new is perceived as difficult or a threat, but given time and a fair evaluation, you will realize that it is not so bad after all.

- *Accept that there will be ups and downs* – No one can hold the same level of motivation forever. Even professional athletes go through slumps, so don't give up over a small set-back. You are allowed to take a break once in a while, and that can even be beneficial over the long run. Just like slipping on your diet, don't beat yourself up over missing a day or two. Take a deep breath and get back to work.

- *Get to know yourself* – Take a long look at what you think you will like and why. Don't try any program that has elements that you know you can't handle or don't have any interest in. Some people love to jog, and others can't stand the idea. There are plenty of choices – types of exercises, when to work out, where to work out, etc. – so make the ones that are most appealing to you. Remember to add music, friends, or anything to make it a better experience.

- *Set a goal and identify rewards* – Think beyond how much weight or inches you will lose or how many crunches you can do, but include how often and how long you want to work out. Include milestones along the way for which you can reward yourself with (no, not an ice cream sundae) a new accessory, CD or DVD, a massage, or some other relatively small 'thank you' gift to yourself. Larger milestones can have larger rewards such as an outfit, a trip, a session with a personal trainer, or anything that is meaningful to you. No matter your incentives, remember that you will have the added bonus of better health!

SIMPLE SUGGESTIONS FOR MAKING EXERCISE MORE FUN

Frame of mind and conscious decision making are important elements that affect the success of any exercise or fitness program. There are also plenty of little touches that can make the process easier and more fun so that you are more likely to stick with it.

- *Post and publicize your goal.* Make sure you see it every day and enlist the help of family and friends to encourage you and help you feel good about your efforts.

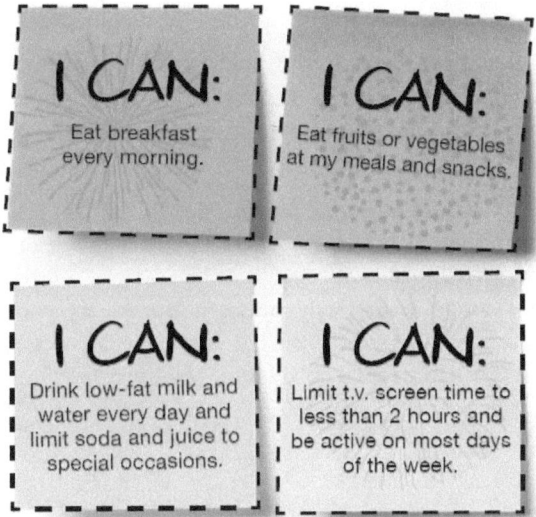

- *Find inspiration.* Don't look at fashion magazines, but instead look at stories about everyday people who have changed their lifestyle. Read anything with a positive message that empowers you.

- *Get enthusiastic.* Think about the positive results you hope to achieve and know that you can do it. Picture how you will look and feel and get excited about the things you will do when you reach your goal. Use that excitement as energy to pull you through your workouts.

- *Work with a partner.* Sharing motivation will help you both on off days, and you can be each other's cheerleader. It's really a great family experience and leads to a lifetime of good behavior when kids learn young.

- *Download a great playlist.* Working out to music you enjoy can make the time pass quickly and give you the rhythm to keep going. Set your activities to the beat so you are comfortable.

- *Allow yourself to feel successful.* Appreciate every improvement you make and congratulate yourself on that success. Each of these little steps leads to another that takes you closer to your milestones and goals. Rate yourself at the end of each week with a gold star or some small reward.

- *Set a low bar.* If you have a hard time getting started, tell yourself it will only be five minutes. Once you get going, you will probably keep going!

- *Make sure your exercise environment is convenient.* Calisthenics and BWT can be done anywhere, but if you live in a cramped apartment, you may have to find another spot.

- *Re-think your choices.* To avoid boredom or burnout, look at your program from time to time and consider making small changes to keep it fun.

- *Learn to listen to your body.* The great thing about improving your fitness level is that you will become more in tune with your body. You will easily recognize that you feel better, but there will be times when your body needs a break. It is important to pay attention to pain or an unusual feeling that comes and goes and fatigue that is not replaced by renewed energy after a workout.

KEEPING A LOG HELPS KEEP YOU ON TRACK

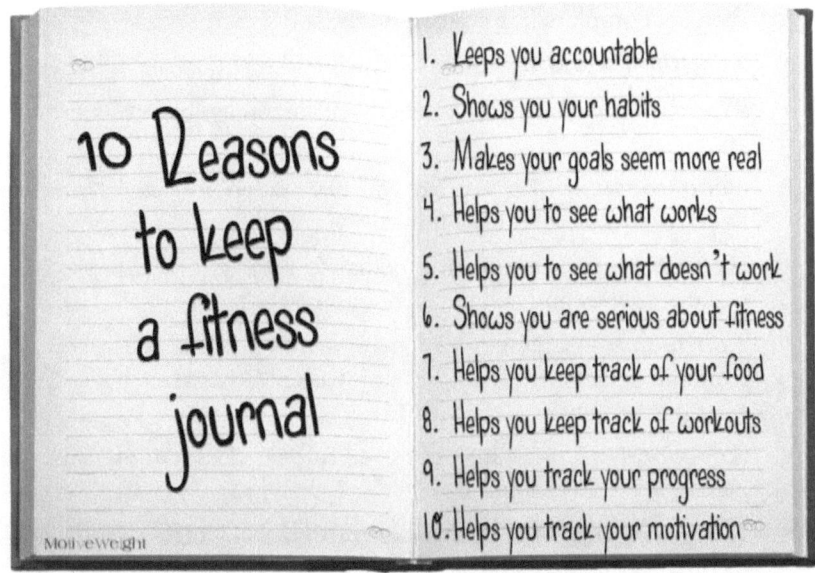

10 Reasons to keep a fitness journal

1. Keeps you accountable
2. Shows you your habits
3. Makes your goals seem more real
4. Helps you to see what works
5. Helps you to see what doesn't work
6. Shows you are serious about fitness
7. Helps you keep track of your food
8. Helps you keep track of workouts
9. Helps you track your progress
10. Helps you track your motivation

Competitive athletes keep fitness logs for specific reasons, such as allowing coaches to devise plans for injury prevention and to make changes that contribute to success and reduce failure. Even non-athletes can benefit from maintaining records about their fitness plans and programs as a means to get fit, stay fit, and determine the best combination of factors for a healthier body and lifestyle.

When setting goals and identifying milestones, it is helpful to have a record showing where you have been and how successfully the program has been working. In order to do that, keeping an exercise journal or log is a great idea. You can simply identify what works and what doesn't, what you like and dislike, and how difficult it may be to perform certain exercises or get past a plateau. You can also use the log as a roadmap to see how far the journey has taken you and how far you have to go to reach your goals.

There are many ways to document your workouts and programs, but there are certain **items that should be included for the most detailed and helpful description.** This is easy to do with a spreadsheet, word document, or even on graph paper in a notebook.

- *Define your fitness goals* – Short, medium, and long-term – at the front of your log, journal, or diary so you can refer to them often to keep you motivated

- *Complete date and time of the workout* – Some days and times are more productive than others

- **Exercise names** – Use a separate column for number of reps and each set completed, distances, times, and weights

- **Length of workout** – Start to finish and rest periods in between

- **Mood** – How you feel physically and mentally, before, during, and after

- **Food consumption** – What you have eaten and when in relation to your workout and how it makes you feel

- **Sleep patterns** – And time demands so it is possible to balance responsibilities and still have enough rest

- **Comments** – Changes you may want to make, ideas you have, something new you learn, or any variable that may have affected your performance

- **Anecdotal notes** – Regarding emotions, distractions, aches and pains, or breakthroughs

- **Body weight, BMI and measurements** – This could be weekly or bi-weekly

- **Include quotes** – Or any type of positive reinforcement that you can refer to quickly for a boost

A number of gyms have their own forms for members to use, and quite a few templates are available online so you just have to fill in the blanks.

Tracking the progression of your fitness efforts is the main reason to maintain a log.

For endurance, there are 3 basic stages:

- **Initial Conditioning Stage** – For non-athletes and those relatively new to exercise, this stage is characterized by an exercise intensity of 40% leading up to 70% of HRmax with a duration of 10 to 20 minutes at a frequency of 2 or 3 times per week. This stage typically lasts for 4 to 5 weeks. The real key is to maintain perfect technical form for the best results.

- **Progressive Performance Stage** – During this stage of increasing difficulty, you will see definite improvement in your overall fitness. You increase HRmax up to 60% to 85% for 3 to 5 sessions lasting 20 to 30 minutes per week. To see this increase in physical performance, your effort has to increase significantly during the 4 to 5 months of this stage but never more than 10% per week. This is for a general level of good fitness – for more specific goals, more time may be required to continue the progressive difficulty of your routine. (See Chapter 8 for more information about progressive training.)

- *Maintenance Stage* – After roughly 6 months of training, you should be able to maintain your fitness level with a program of exercise 3 times per week working at 70% to 85% HRmax for 30 to 45 minutes per session.

Weight resistance training programs for general fitness are based on the performance of at least 7 to 10 different exercises that target all the major muscle groups twice per week, working to muscle fatigue. You should maintain the best technique possible for 8 to 12 reps utilizing full range of motion, control on both the concentric (lifting) and eccentric (lowering) phases of each exercise, and normal breathing patterns. Depending on your goals, the basic rule is to increase resistance for greater muscle mass and increase reps for definition and endurance.

An important factor to keep in mind is that there is no set 'prescription' for improvement. There are simply too many individual elements that determine one person's success over another's to provide a 'one size fits all' program. Newbies will be able to significantly increase the percentage of intensity as compared to athletes because they have so much room for improvement. For example, if you do 2 reps this week and 4 reps next week, that's a lot easier than 20 this week and 40 next week although both figures are simply doubled. Other considerations are age, general fitness, fat vs. muscle mass, starting weight, gender, and even the length of arms and legs relative to overall body size (since it all goes back to geometry and physics)!

CHAPTER 5

How The Body Creates
And Uses Energy

In order for the body to function properly – in fact, to function at all – it requires energy. Even at rest, energy reserves burn to promote healing, growth and maintain cellular function. For optimal performance, it is important to have a steady supply of nutrients and a well-tuned metabolism so that the cells can process the stored fuel and provide energy for muscular exertion.

The true benefit of exercise is that it regulates and enhances the body's use of oxygen and nutrients for more efficient delivery. In other words, a combination of physiological and neurological processes that are stimulated to work not only during a workout but also afterwards to return the body to *homeostasis* (the efforts of the body to maintain stability or, simply put, a happy medium).

THE CONNECTION BETWEEN OXYGEN AND ENERGY

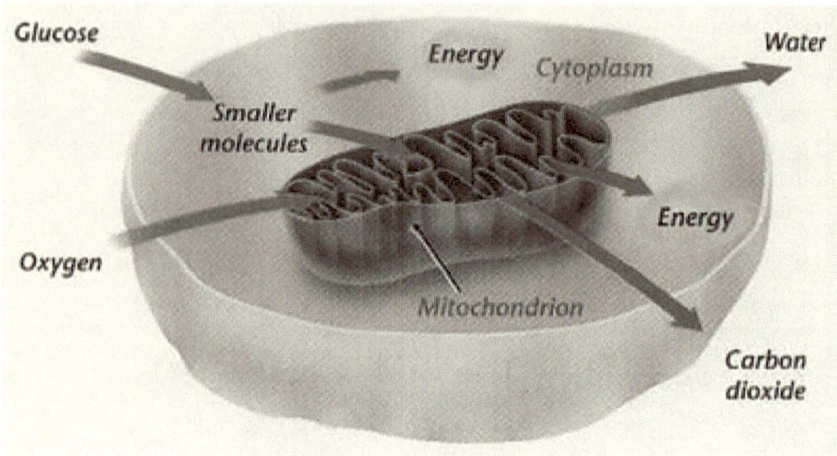

Without oxygen, the cells in the human body begin to die. This is true after as little as 60 seconds of strenuous exercise if there is no transfer of oxygen to the cells. Oxygen is the catalyst behind the conversion of stored fuel in the body into useful energy, and every day, all day this conversion constantly continues. The good news is that exercise improves this function.

This type of respiration takes place within the cells in the tiny components called the *mitochondria*. It is the conversion of fat or sugar stored in the cell that creates the compound *Adenosine Triphosphate* (ATP), which is the actual fuel that keeps the cells active and that the muscles burn to perform their functions. Without enough oxygen to stimulate the conversion process, lactic acid builds up and this can lead to muscle spasms.

Through regular exercise, especially when the body is pushed to its limits repeatedly after very brief rest periods, the mitochondria actually increase in number and density. This means that the body is capable of producing even more energy faster to fuel the added demands of the muscles. After intense workouts, the body continues to burn energy so that the cells can replace their stores of nutrients. In other words, **the effects of exercise last much longer than just the actual workout**.

Sugar and fat are the two sources of stored energy in all cells. Sugar is easier to burn, but fat provides twice as much energy. When the body has used up the readily available glucose in the cells, it has to turn to burning fat. That is when weight loss becomes easier – getting rid of the built-up fat to fuel the body and promote even more movement. As the cells improve the efficient conversion of fuel to energy, they also increase their use of oxygen and provide better elimination of carbon dioxide and other waste products.

A tremendous variety of nutrients from different food sources is required by the cells to maintain proper, efficient functioning. Different compounds are responsible for the cell membrane, the nucleus, the transfer of energy, and internal communication. When any of these elements is jeopardized, the result can be disastrous, leading to many different diseases and conditions. Whole foods that are not contaminated with toxins are the best source of the appropriate building blocks to maintain cellular integrity.

AEROBIC VS. ANAEROBIC EXERCISES

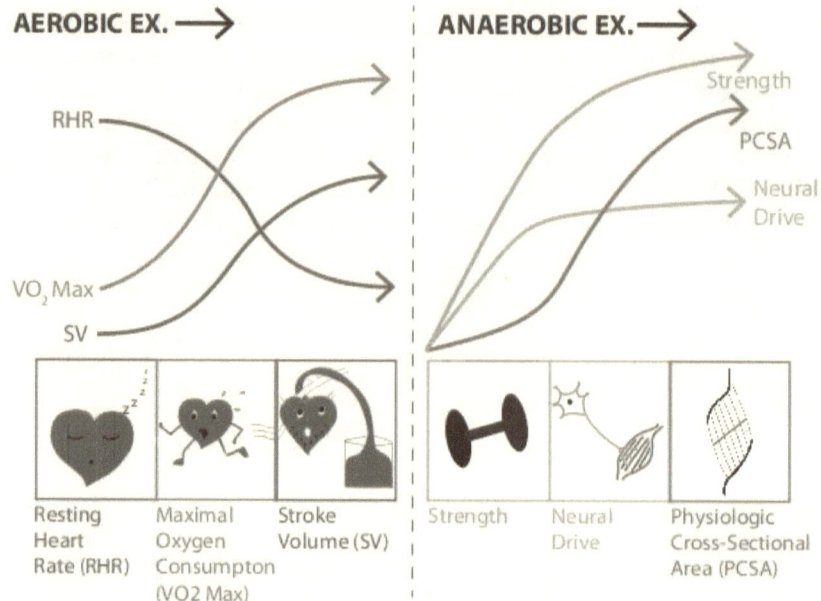

Most people who have participated in some sort of exercise have heard the term 'aerobics.' *Aerobic exercise* is generally moderately to fast paced and is designed to raise the heart rate over a period of time. Aerobics is considered endurance training. Glycogen is, as well as some fats are, burned for energy, and increased respiration removes carbon dioxide efficiently. Because this activity takes place over time, lactic acid is not usually able to build up. Typical aerobic activities include running, biking, and swimming.

Anaerobic exercise is quite different because it involves intense bursts of activity such as sprinting or weight lifting that demand high energy burn. This depletes glycogen quickly, and the buildup of lactic acid due to the lack of oxygen results in 'hitting the wall' – a state of discomfort and exhaustion. The importance of anaerobic activity is the increase of lean muscle mass that allows the body to burn more calories, even when the body is at rest. It is also what weight lifters and body builders aim for to increase the mass of specific muscles.

Performing calisthenics and bodyweight training gives you the opportunity to mix aerobic and anaerobic activities for the best overall fitness. This use of both exercise styles is called *interval training* and has been the standard routine for all sorts of athletes for many years.

WHERE DO CARBOHYDRATES FIT IN?

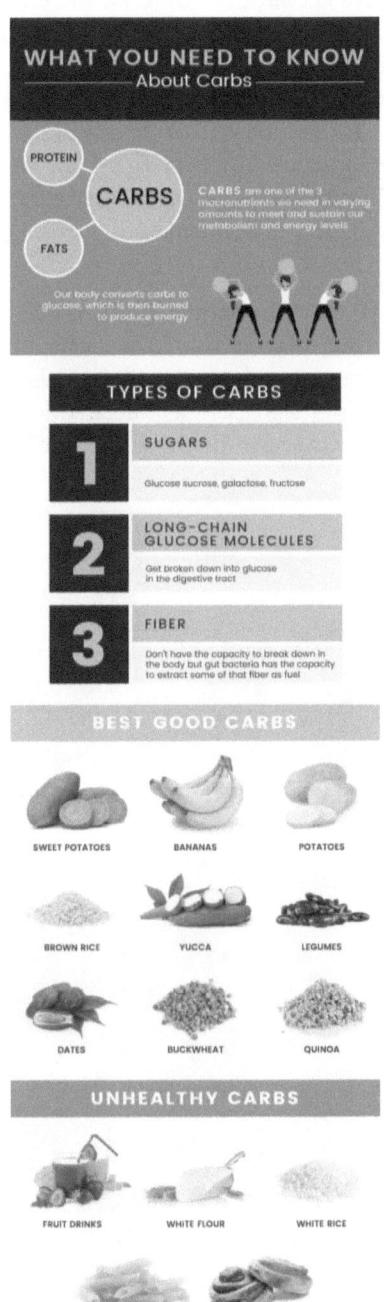

For anyone considering weight loss, the key word is **carbohydrates**. The fact is that carbohydrates account for most of the energy that is used by the body and are the product stored in muscle cells and the liver in the form of glycogen. Most people don't use up the glycogen stores in their body in regular exercise workouts. With up to 4,000 calories to burn at one time, it takes intense activity to get past that threshold. Making sure that the carbohydrates you consume are not 'easy fixes' like candy bars is one way to prevent the accumulation of fat since sugars are burned up quickly but leave the other carbohydrates that are not used for glycogen replacement to be stored as fat.

Not only are the types of carbohydrates you consume important but the overall quality of your diet plays a role in the efficient functioning of cells. Fats and proteins are crucial for cellular shape and activity and phytonutrients from plants also play a crucial role in supplying nutrients. Nutrition and diet are discussed in the next chapter in greater detail.

BALANCE FOOD AND ACTIVITY FOR FITNESS

Energy can also be thought of as calories and that is a word any dieter knows. The equation is quite simple – **the calories you take in must equal the calories you burn up** through cellular and physical activity if you do not want to gain weight. The body uses energy for its own maintenance, but beyond those needs, without physical exertion, extra calories add up to weight gain.

Men and women have different caloric needs, as do children when compared to adults and the elderly. As early as age 4, males require roughly 200 more calories a day than females, and at puberty, that changes to 400 calories. For both sexes, though, the overall calorie requirement begins to drop by 200 calories at age 30, so consuming the same amount of food you always have will only add weight. At any stage of life, however, for both men and women, the difference between higher calorie intake and lower output leads to the same problem – being overweight.

Identifying your activity level is an important step in determining how many calories your body needs for basic functioning. **There are 4 levels of activity** defined as:

- *Sedentary* – Light physical activity encountered in daily life. This means you have a sit-down job, park close to your destinations to avoid walking, and don't engage in exercise.

- *Moderate* – Added to the typical cellular life activities, you may also perform the exercise equivalent of walking anywhere from 1.5 to 3 miles **each** day at a slow pace.

- *Active* – A step up from moderate, you perform the equivalent of a 5- to 10-mile walk at a slow pace as well as the daily cellular life activities **every** day (burning 600-1,000 calories).

- *Very active* – Planned exercise that is equal to walking more than 10 miles **per day** (burning more than 1,000 calories).

Think of **balancing your energy and calories** the same way you balance a bank account. If you are anticipating a high calorie intake event such as a party, burn more calories ahead of time to compensate. If you know that you will be restricted in your time or ability to exercise, cut back on your calorie consumption.

For dieting or weight loss, the equation is just as simple. You need to burn up more calories than you consume. At the beginning, it is better to add some physical activity so that your body gets used to the idea of burning calories. Once you have revved up your metabolism, cut back on the calories, starting with unhealthy sugars and fats. You don't want your metabolism to respond to a cutback of calories by slowing down! That just makes the job harder! This is a problem that women face more than men due to the inherent biological need to reserve nutrients to continue to care for children in times of famine. That is why it seems that men can lose weight faster – they actually do!

Given the fact that a pound of fat contains 3,500 calories, it follows that a reduction of 500 calories a day over the course of a week should result in the loss of 1 pound of body weight. Combine diet and an activity increase of 500 calories, and that pound would come off in half the time. That amount of energy burn requires at least moderate activity every day, each day of the week.

HOW TO CALCULATE YOUR CALORIES

Basal Metabolic Rate (BMR) is the number of calories you would burn with NO activity.

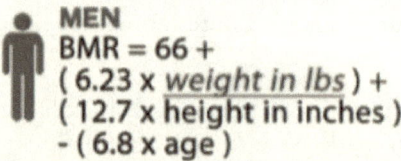

MEN
BMR = 66 +
(6.23 x *weight in lbs*) +
(12.7 x height in inches)
- (6.8 x age)

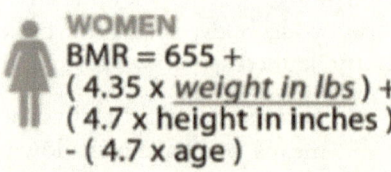

WOMEN
BMR = 655 +
(4.35 x *weight in lbs*) +
(4.7 x height in inches)
- (4.7 x age)

(TIP: use __Lean Body weight__ (% body fat x weight in lbs) if possible)

YOUR TARGET DAILY CALORIE NEEDS

1. Little or no exercise: BMR x 1.2

2. Light Exercise/sports 1-3 days/week: BMR x 1.375

3. Medium Exercise/sports 3-5 days/week: BMR x 1.55

4. Hard Exercise/sports 6-7 days a week: BMR x 1.725

5. Intense exercise/sports, physical job or twice/day training): BMR x 1.9

SLEEP IS A KEY INGREDIENT FOR HEALTH AND FITNESS

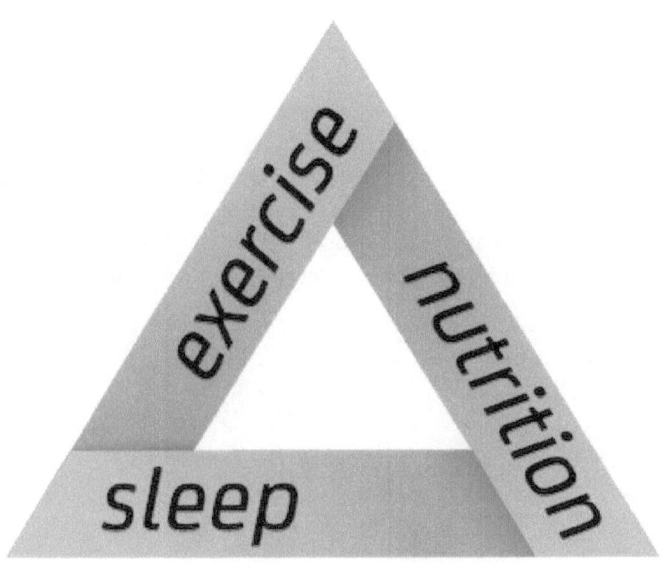

It is during periods of rest that the body repairs and replenishes itself, both physically and mentally. Since sleep affects the endocrine system of the body, which regulates hormones, the lack of sleep prevents the appropriate messages regarding hunger and fullness from getting to the brain. This results in over-eating and the craving for carbohydrate-rich snacks, especially later in the evening. The fat cells are less sensitive to insulin, and growth- and thyroid-stimulating hormones are affected with the likely end result of diabetes and other metabolic disruptions.

Activity, particularly regular workouts, forces more oxygen and nutrients into the brain due to the increased blood flow. This helps improve mental function and makes you feel more alert and able to focus. The regular, repeated increase in blood flow trains the brain to expect the changes, and this is believed to help protect against problems like Alzheimer's or Parkinson's disease or even stroke.

When the body is well rested and engages in activity, the mitochondria consume oxygen efficiently to convert glycogen and fat to fuel. Intense exercise leads to mitochondrial biogenesis, the creation of new mitochondria, and the whole process is enhanced. Other beneficial chemical reactions also take place more easily such as the production of Human Growth Hormone (HGH), which stimulates fat-burning as well as muscle building and strengthening and the increase in catecholamine, which stimulates the conversion of fat into useable energy.

Stress is both a psychological as well as a physiological factor that affects and is affected by rest. While exercise is actually the addition of stress to the body, the release of endorphins (feel-good hormones), dopamine, and serotonin can help combat emotional stress. After exercise, the mood is elevated, the flow of oxygen through the body is enhanced and rest can come easier in order to provide the regeneration of your body and spirit.

Just like a fine-tuned piece of machinery, you get the most out of your body and your life when there is an appropriate balance of healthy food, rest, and exercise.

CHAPTER 6

The Role Of Nutrition In
Weight Loss And Management

Nutrition is really a simple concept, but unfortunately, many people don't pay attention to the basic rules. Processed, packaged, and fast food have become the norm, and the healthy nutrition of whole foods has been lost to a large extent through modern forms of handling. This has undermined the function of the human body since fiber and many of the necessary minerals have been stripped away from the foods we eat. Convenience has many people overloading on carbs and fats, and the result is an ever-increasing waistline and sluggish feeling.

UNDERSTANDING WHAT THE BODY NEEDS

Everyone has heard the term, '*a well-balanced diet*,' but what does that really mean? The body needs food from a wide range of sources to provide the daily requirements for healthy functioning such as:

- Proteins from fish, fowl, lean meats, and nuts
- Vegetables and fruits
- Whole grains
- Dairy
- Healthy fats and oils
- Limited amounts of refined grains, potatoes, white rice (carbohydrates!)
- Only minimal amounts of other items such as salt, sugar, and processed foods

This has been illustrated in a variety of forms – the food pyramid and a divided plate – to show the appropriate proportions of each of these types of foods.

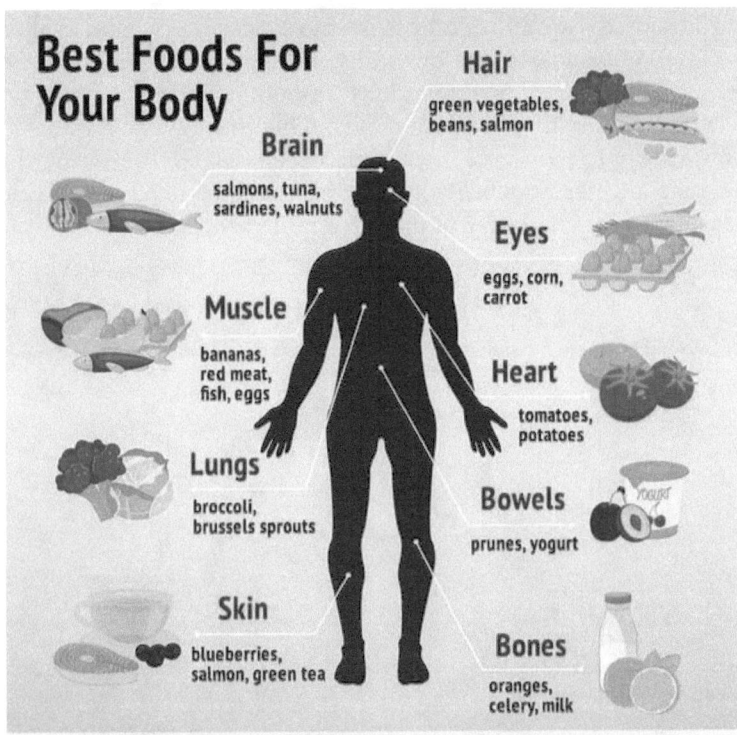

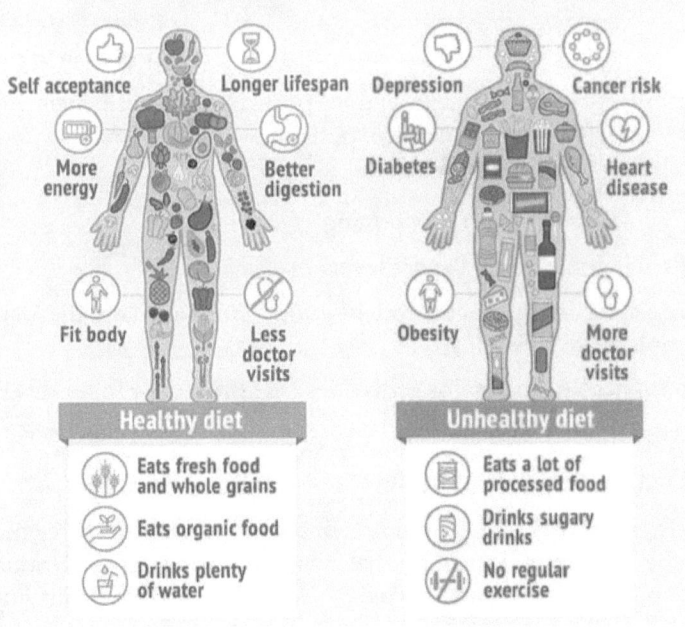

Dieting is usually a bad idea because most people go about it all wrong. When someone decides to go on a diet, the path tends to be an extreme change, and this causes a tremendous amount of stress on the body to which it responds with drastic measures. This means that the metabolism will slow down to conserve the available energy in the event that the 'famine' lasts a while. So while you are consuming less and less calories, the body is using fewer and fewer of them for basic functions.

THE VICIOUS DIET CYCLE

REPEAT

overweight

decrease in calories

DIET

FEAST RESPONSE

- Reduced metabolic rate
- Loss of muscle
- Regain weight from fat

increase in calories

FAMINE RESPONSE

- Lose weight from lean muscle and fat
- Reduced metabolic rate
- Increase in fat storage

FALL OFF

Even cutting out carbohydrates causes problems because there are other functions these complex chains perform besides 'making you fat.' **Carbohydrates are needed for**:

- Cellular growth and functioning
- Regulation of blood sugar levels
- Assisting in the regulation of blood pressure and the control of cholesterol levels
- Supply of nutrients for probiotics that promote proper digestion
- Absorption of calcium
- Fuel for the CNS and brain

Particularly when you are planning on starting an exercise regimen, you should take a careful look at what you are using to fuel your body. **Endurance athletes 'load carbs'** – in other words, consume large amounts of carbohydrates for the glucose they will supply throughout athletic performance. Unlike these athletes, though, most people consume more than enough carbs for their exercise needs. Some carbs such as processed sugar and wheat products should be avoided or limited, but there are many other healthy sources of carbohydrates. The most important consideration is not necessarily the amount but the source of the carbohydrates.

Eating a **diet extremely high in protein can also be unhealthy** for a number of reasons. Since the burning of body fat and available protein causes a buildup of *ketones* (the product of burning these fuel sources), this can lead to an imbalance in the body's chemistry resulting in acidosis, unpleasant bad breath and body odor, and even a coma. There is a diet program based on this principle, but it must be monitored carefully. Muscle tissue is made up of protein so the body can actually start to burn its own tissues for fuel when there is not enough available protein for muscle maintenance. The limitation of other types of foods can bring about constipation and diseases due to vitamin insufficiencies.

Instead of looking at a diet as the need to cut out certain foods, it should be looked at as a healthy plan for supplying *all* the nutrients the body needs in the right proportions. With the addition of higher quality fuel, your body will function better, and you will feel better.

SELECTING A HEALTHY DIET

There are many different sources that describe the 'ideal' diet but the **basic recommendations** can be broken down as follows:

1. Whole grains (cereal, bread, pasta, and rice) and other carbs such as barley, cornmeal, beans, flax, and quinoa – 6-11 servings each day

2. Fresh, clean fruits and vegetables – 5-9 servings each day (raw is best for many of these choices)

3. Dairy products such as milk, cheese, and yogurt – 2-4 servings each day

4. Protein from fish, fowl, lean meats, eggs, nuts, and beans – 2-3 servings each day

5. Healthy fats and oils – monounsaturated fats such as olive, sunflower, peanut, and sesame oil and avocados, olives, and a variety of nuts such as peanuts, hazelnuts, almonds, pecans, cashews, and macadamia nuts

6. Very limited amounts of potatoes, white rice, and refined, processed grains (**This** is what most people think of as carbohydrates, and they should be eliminated!)

7. Minimal amounts of other items including salt, sugar, processed foods, and alcohol

15 FOODS THAT BOOST YOUR METABOLISM

GRAPEFRUIT GREEN TEA YOGURT ALMONDS COFFEE

TURKEY APPLES SPINACH BEANS JALAPENOS

BROCCOLI CURRY CINNAMON SOYMILK OATMEAL

Another important issue for people who need to limit their food intake to control calories is **portion control**. What you see on most plates is significantly more than an appropriate portion! In some cases, one meal may contain more calories than are needed in a whole day!

- One serving of meat is 3 oz. – roughly the size of a bar of soap or a checkbook.
- Cooked pasta (1/2 cup) is the size of a fist.
- Bread, waffles, or pancakes should be about the size of a CD case.
- 4 Cheese cubes the size of dice make up one serving.
- Fruit and fresh veggies (about 1 cup) should be the size of a baseball or tennis ball.

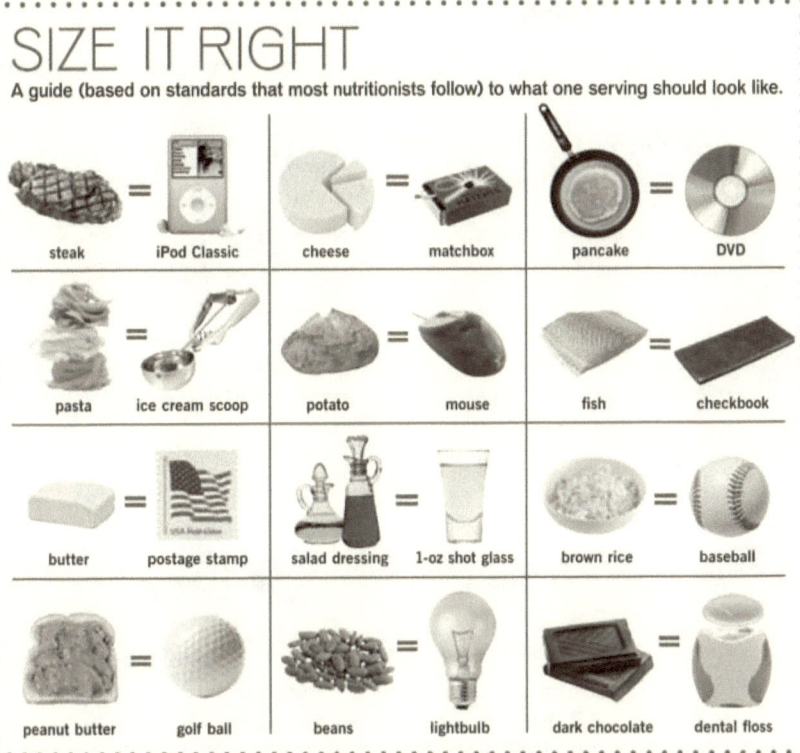

SIZE IT RIGHT
A guide (based on standards that most nutritionists follow) to what one serving should look like.

steak	= iPod Classic	cheese	= matchbox	pancake	= DVD
pasta	= ice cream scoop	potato	= mouse	fish	= checkbook
butter	= postage stamp	salad dressing	= 1-oz shot glass	brown rice	= baseball
peanut butter	= golf ball	beans	= lightbulb	dark chocolate	= dental floss

The best way to serve appropriate portion sizes is to measure the food. That is quite problematic for most people, however, so one way to get around that is to measure basic portions with water and pour it into your usual dishes. It will come as quite a surprise when you see that what you pour as a bowl of cereal could actually amount to 2, 3, or even more servings! Getting used to the size of different portions in relation to your own plates and bowls will help you cut down the amount of food you eat and reduce caloric intake. Another trick is to serve yourself a typical portion, remove half, and put it aside as another meal.

THE QUESTION OF SUPPLEMENTS

In an effort to increase energy, overcome stress, and optimize physical performance, many people believe that it is necessary to take nutritional supplements. For the most part, however, experts agree that eating a well-balanced diet is all that is needed for you to meet your energy requirements. With the exception of pregnant women and older adults who may benefit from supplements such as folic acid and vitamin C and calcium, respectively, your daily dietary intake should supply everything you need.

Fresh, whole foods that are produced as organically as possible contribute to your health in 3 major ways:

1. Provide a wider range of micronutrients for overall better nutrition

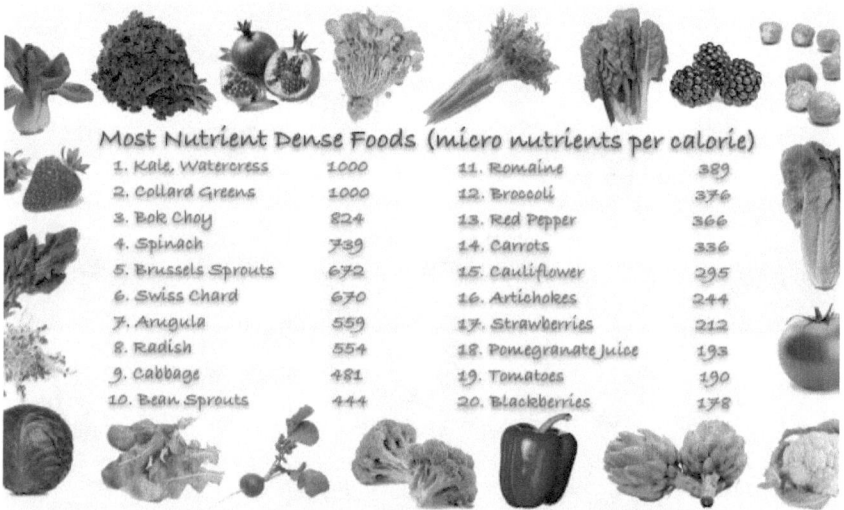

Most Nutrient Dense Foods (micro nutrients per calorie)

1. Kale, Watercress	1000	11. Romaine	389
2. Collard Greens	1000	12. Broccoli	376
3. Bok Choy	824	13. Red Pepper	366
4. Spinach	739	14. Carrots	336
5. Brussels Sprouts	672	15. Cauliflower	295
6. Swiss Chard	670	16. Artichokes	244
7. Arugula	559	17. Strawberries	212
8. Radish	554	18. Pomegranate Juice	193
9. Cabbage	481	19. Tomatoes	190
10. Bean Sprouts	444	20. Blackberries	178

2. Provide the necessary dietary fiber for healthy digestion
3. Provide additional compounds such as phytochemicals and antioxidants, which work within the body to protect against a number of diseases such as cancer, heart disease, and diabetes

There are other experts however who claim that even eating what is considered to be a well-balanced diet is not sufficient since the foods we eat come from nutrient-depleted soils or are picked early and force-ripened. The way food is prepared can also reduce the value of the nutrients you would expect to receive. Canned and processed foods have lost much of their inherent nutritional value and further cooking only reduces the level more. Additionally, when the skins of fruits and vegetables are removed, some of the highest concentrations of the product's nutritional value are lost.

So what is the public supposed to do? If you are concerned about your health (and since you are reading this book, you must be!), you should consult a nutritionist or your primary healthcare professional for the best advice. Beyond a multivitamin and perhaps a fiber supplement, different products can have unexpected side effects with one another or with prescription medication you may be taking. Let a professional help with the decision to add any other nutritional supplements to improve your physical and mental performance to avoid complications.

For body builders and hard-core athletes, protein supplements may be helpful right after intense workouts. For anyone else, there should be adequate protein in the diet, and if more protein is needed, it can come from the addition of some nuts, lean meat, a glass of skim or low-fat milk, or one of the other many protein sources as a snack. As with any supplement, **protein powders and shakes** are made from a variety of sources and have any number of additives, much of which can be carbohydrates. The best options include *whey* and *casein*, which come from milk and soy which is plant-based.

Building muscle mass involves eating more of the right kinds of foods, especially those high in protein. Lean, grass-fed beef, chicken, fish, eggs, and dairy products are key sources of protein, but there are also other foods that play important roles in overall muscle mass. Brown rice, quinoa, whole grains, and oatmeal provide a variety of nutrients containing essential amino acids, help control insulin production, boost growth hormone levels, and help you feel full longer. Fruits and vegetables are also quite important and among the most beneficial are apples, oranges, beets, spinach and other dark green, leafy vegetables, tomatoes, and broccoli. Whey powder is a great supplement and can be used for a drink after a workout.

Eating smaller meals more frequently (or at 3 least moderate meals with 3 healthy snacks) is the ideal way to keep the body fueled and provide all the essential nutrients for muscle growth and maintenance. In each of these six 'meals,' include a bit of protein; for mid-morning and mid-afternoon snacks, some yogurt and fruit, a smoothie with protein powder, low fat milk and fruit or some fruit, whole wheat bread or crackers and peanut butter offer an energy boost and muscle-building protein.

High-Protein Snacks for Energy

These protein-rich foods offer satiety and a boost of energy without sugar and sweeteners.

- Cottage cheese
- Plain yogurt
- Kefir
- "Natural" cheese
- Nuts
- Unsweetened nut butters
- Dried edamame
- Chia seeds soaked in water
- Soy nuts
- Hard-boiled eggs
- Roasted pumpkin and squash seeds
- Cured meats (jerky, salami, etc.)
- Hummus with veggies
- Bean dip with veggies

THE BODY ALSO NEEDS PLENTY OF WATER

Water is the primary component of our bodies, and it needs to be replenished regularly. During strenuous exercise when the body sweats, fluid is lost rather quickly and must be replaced. For intense workouts, it can add up to anywhere from 2 to 3 gallons!

Water has several important functions in the body:

- It helps to regulate body temperature.
- It provides fluid to the blood to aid in the transport of oxygen and nutrients.
- It flushes out cellular wastes and toxins.
- It enhances the digestive process and kidney function.

Sports drinks are very popular, but there are those who believe that plain water is all the body needs for adequate hydration. For most individuals who are working out for less than an hour at a moderate rate, that is probably true, but there are advantages to consuming products with added electrolytes and carbohydrates when intense or long-lasting activity takes place.

Too much water can actually be counter-productive in that it triggers the kidneys to release excess fluid and dehydration can result. The sodium in sports drinks compensates for the salt lost through sweat and is important because it helps the body retain water and directs the fluids to the blood stream and appropriate muscles. Carbohydrates provide an easy source of energy for cells that are tiring, giving them a boost for longer endurance.

Another word of caution about the type of beverage you choose to address hydration: you should avoid drinking a sugary beverage because the sudden flood of sugar is burned as fuel much more easily than fat or protein, but when the sugar is gone, the body takes a while to adjust to the change, leading to what is called a 'sugar crash.' Carbonated beverages should also be avoided because of the discomfort that can result from the gas and the possibility of developing cramps and diarrhea.

CLEANSING THE BODY

Detoxification is a trendy topic with a lot of pros and cons. Drastic measures such as colonic flushes or special diets with periods of fasting are not considered to be really necessary, but attention should be paid to the idea of helping the body remove toxins. This is especially true when beginning a diet and exercise plan since many toxins are stored in fat. When the fat is broken down, these toxins are released into the system and this sudden rush can cause feelings of fatigue, muscle soreness, and even nausea. A healthy diet and the increase in metabolic activity due to exercise will keep the detoxification pathways clear for better functioning.

There are several **ways in which the body removes toxic elements**:

- Digestive process
- Kidneys (to the bladder and elimination through the urine)
- Liver (filters the blood)
- Lymphatic system
- Respiratory system
- Skin (through sweat)

One way to get more enjoyment out of your food and aid in the detox process is to **add a variety of herbs and spices**. *Anise, Basil, Burdock, Cilantro, Cinnamon, Cayenne, Cloves, Cumin, Garlic, Ginger, Ginseng, Licorice, Milk Thistle, Mint, Nutmeg, Oregano, Rosemary, Sage, Schisandra, Thyme,* and *Turmeric* all provide benefits to digestion.

In order to maintain a steady supply of nutrients, it is suggested that you add a few healthy snacks that include a small portion of lean protein or nuts mid-morning and mid-afternoon. Green tea is a healthy option as opposed to coffee, and adding some lemon wedges or juice to water benefits a wide assortment of issues in the body.

Once you begin a healthier lifestyle, the process becomes easier and easier. A proper diet provides better physical function and more energy so that exercise is less of a struggle and more exercise provides more energy and a greater utilization of oxygen and nutrients that lead to weight loss. When you feel good, you will continue to do the things that support that state of being so you are more likely to continue eating properly and exercising regularly.

CHAPTER 7

Essential Calisthenics And
Bodyweight Exercises

Done properly, calisthenics and bodyweight exercises can help you achieve virtually any fitness goal. After all, this was how it has been done for thousands of years! The important thing to realize is that **it is not necessarily how many reps or sets you can do as much as it is the precision with which you perform them**. Just like having the tires balanced on the car, utilizing the correct form works the muscles for their optimum efficiency.

A key element in performing calisthenics correctly is your body's ability to move through space in a controlled manner. There are receptors in the joints as well as the sense of balance in the inner ear that help us identify where our body parts are in relation to one another and the floor. Learning the proper way to perform an exercise and repeating that movement over and over helps train the CNS. It enables the coordination of all the muscles flexing and relaxing to become automatic. This is how a baseball pitcher perfects a pitch or a golfer masters a putt.

Beyond simply exercising for general fitness and weight loss, perfecting the steps of these basic exercises allows anyone to train for advanced athletics, increased strength, and well-defined muscle mass.

BEGIN WITH THE BASICS

Although there are literally hundreds of different options that qualify as calisthenics or bodyweight exercises, the basics are where they all begin. Here are **12 simple exercises** that can get anyone in better shape and improve cardiovascular function. Try working out **at least twice a week** but not more than 4 times until you build up your strength and stamina.

Focus on perfecting your form so that each exercise is performed correctly:

- *Begin with 8 reps of each* (except where noted) *for a set* and slowly increase by one or two reps every week or two. This should last 6 to 8 weeks or slightly longer for beginners.

- When you are comfortable with 12 reps and can maintain the correct form, *drop back to 8 reps but do 2 sets*.

- Continue adding reps until you reach 12 and then *start over with 8 reps but with 3 sets*.

Another option for improving your workout is to **gradually add new exercises** to the group of basics. From the 12 basics, you can create many variations that work different muscles and add more of a challenge to your workout. Chapter 9, "Amping Up the Basic Workout," provides tips and instructions for more advanced forms of these basic exercises for true muscle mass and strength building.

PUSH UP PROGRESSIONS
FROM BEGINNER TO ADVANCED

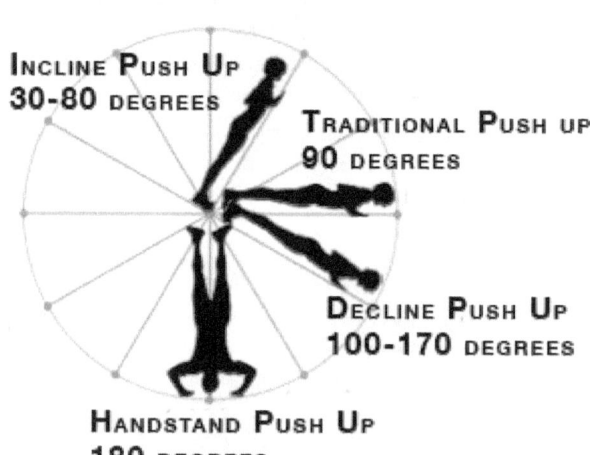

INCLINE PUSH UP
30-80 DEGREES

TRADITIONAL PUSH UP
90 DEGREES

DECLINE PUSH UP
100-170 DEGREES

HANDSTAND PUSH UP
180 DEGREES

Remember that **ALL workouts should include a warm-up and a cool down**. These two aspects are vital, but also quite simple. Simply stretching and running in place or something similar for 2 to 3 minutes is all it takes but can make the difference between a great workout and a painful one.

Bridges

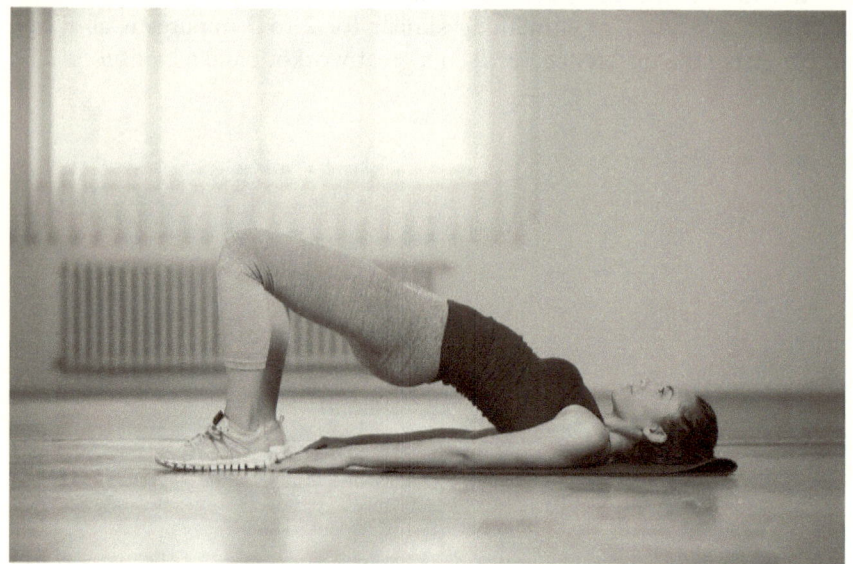

- Lay flat on your back. Extend your arms along your sides. Place the bottoms of your feet on the floor and bend your knees.

- Keep your abs contracted as you raise your hips up from the floor.

- Hold for 3-5 seconds and return to the floor for 1 rep. (Flex your feet so that your weight rests on your heels for some extra pull.)

Burpees (Squat Jump Thrusts)

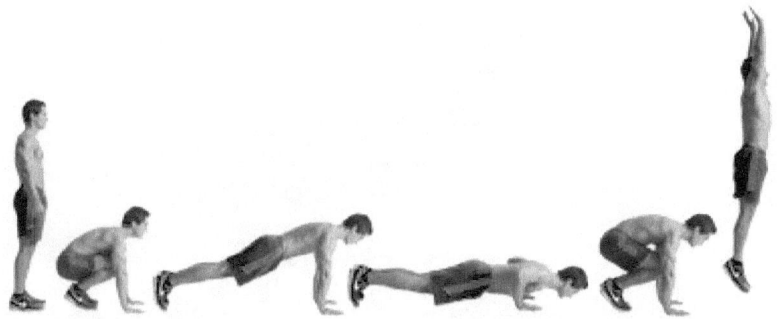

- Stand up straight with abs engaged and shoulders back.
- Lower to a squat position with your hands in front of your feet.
- Balance on your hands with your arms straight and thrust your legs back into the plank.
- Jump to return to a squat, then stand up (jump up) to complete 1 rep.

Crunches

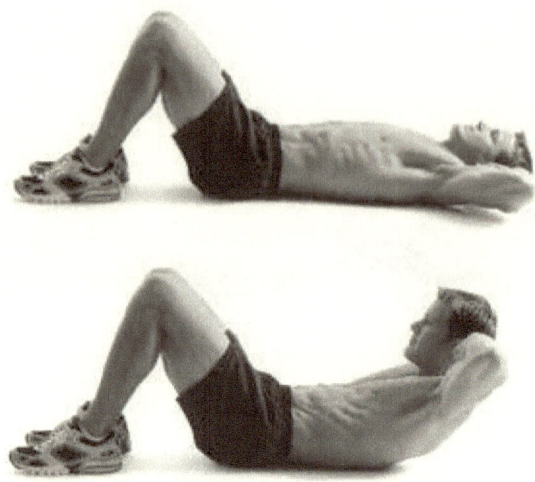

- Lay down on your back. Bend your knees into 90-degree angles. Rest your feet on the floor.

- Your arms can be crossed against your chest or rested at your sides, or place your hands at the back of your head.

- Engage your abs and exhale as you lift your shoulder blades off the floor.

- Do not strain your neck or crunch your head forward. Look up at the ceiling and simply move your rib cage towards your hips.

Jumping Jacks

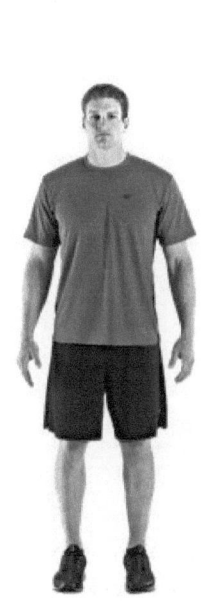 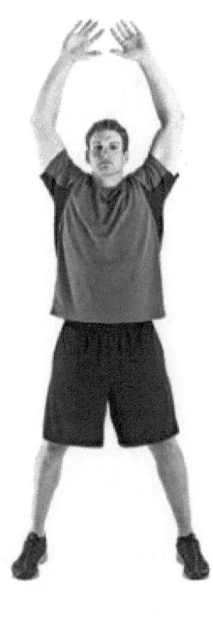

- Stand with your feet close. Let your arms rest.
- Jump up while inhaling, spreading feet and clapping your hands overhead.
- In a continuous movement, jump up again to return your feet to the start and your arms back at your sides.
- Keep your abs tight and your back straight.
- Perform 20 to 30 reps for a set, maintaining a comfortable pace.

Lunges

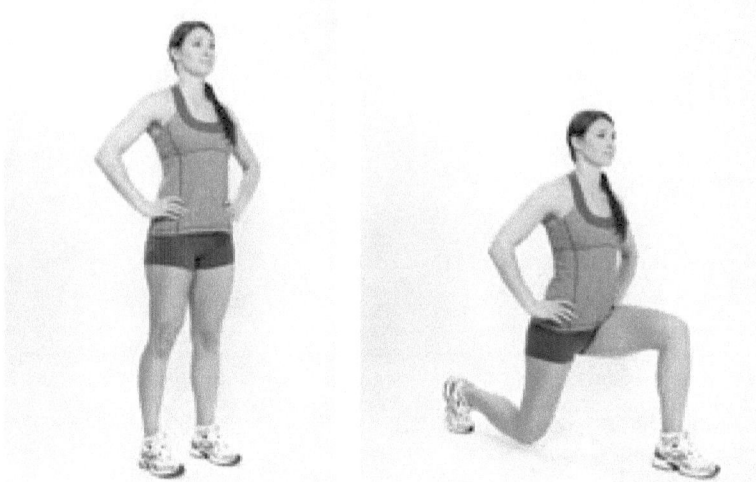

- Stand up straight with feet hip width apart.
- Maintaining an erect posture with your head in line with your spine, take a large step forward bringing your back heel off the floor.
- Lower your body so that both knees are bent at roughly 90 degrees.
- Keep your abs tight and breathe deeply from the diaphragm.
- Push off the front foot and return to a standing position.
- Switch legs and repeat for 1 rep.

Oblique Leg Lifts

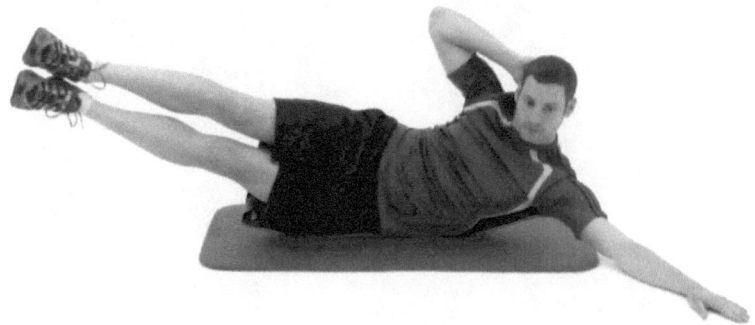

- Lay on the floor on your side, rest your legs on top of each other. Your lower arm can be extended for balance or bent in front of your body, while the upper arm can rest along your side or over your waist.

- Lift your upper leg toward your shoulder and bring that shoulder forward, trying to bring your ribs and hips together.

- Lower your leg and relax your shoulder for 1 rep.

- Switch sides to complete one set.

For more of a challenge, lift both legs together.

Planks

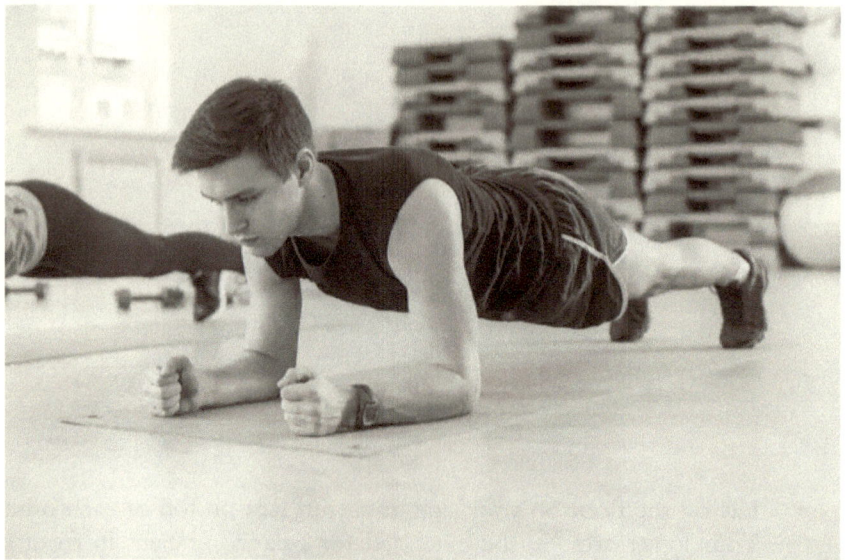

- Begin in a raised push-up position, arms shoulder width apart.
- Lower yourself so that your forearms are flat, hands out in front with palms down, and elbows under your shoulders.
- Maintaining a tight core and flat back with your eyes on the floor, hold the position until you feel the 'burn,' about 20 to 30 seconds.
- Relax and repeat for a total of 3 reps.

Pull Ups and Chin Ups

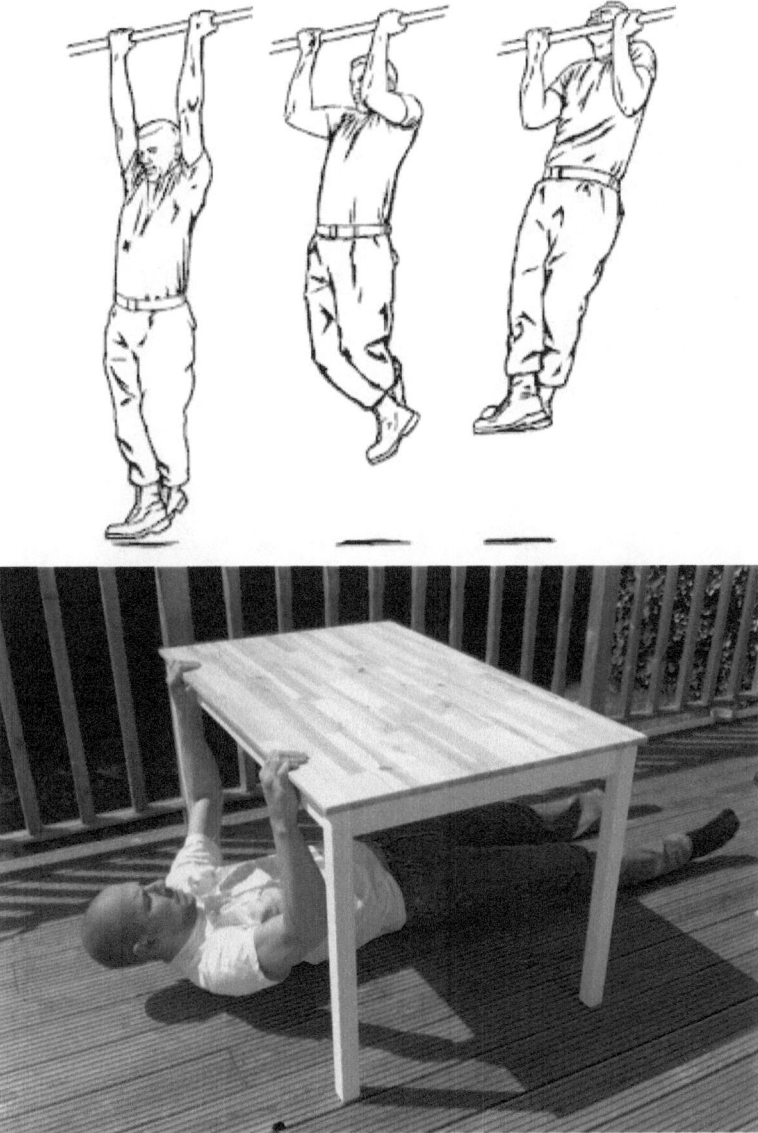

- From the dead hang position, with hands at shoulder width and turning palms outward, raise your body until your chin passes the bar.

- With control, lower yourself for 6 to 8 reps.

- Be sure not to kick or swing.

Negative Pull Ups

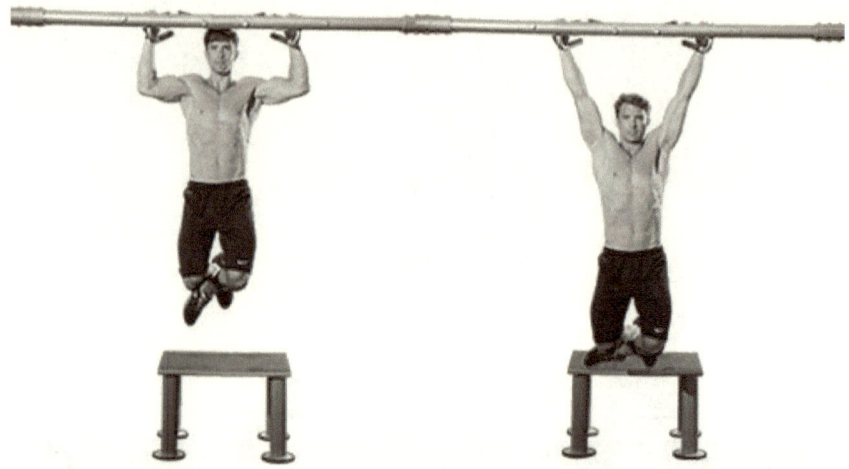

- If you can't accomplish a regular pull-up, start building those muscles with flexed arm hangs.

- Get into the pull-up position, chin above the bar, with the help of a stool or workout partner, and hold that position as long as possible.

- For negative pull-ups, get into the chin-up position with the help of a stool or workout partner and lower yourself as slowly as possible.

These exercises work with gravity and help you build up muscle and grip strength. Reverse hand grip (palms facing you) for chin-ups.

Push Ups

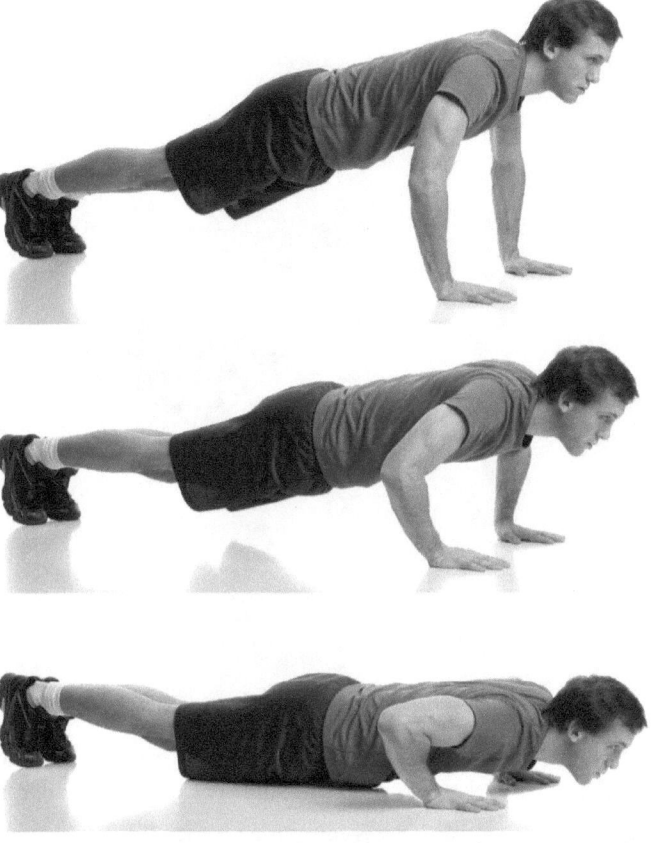

- Lie on your belly, elbows in tight to your sides, and hands shoulder width apart on the floor.

- Extend your arms, keeping your back straight, your abs engaged, and your head in line with your back.

- Bend your elbows and lower yourself as far as possible without touching the floor for 1 rep.

Squats

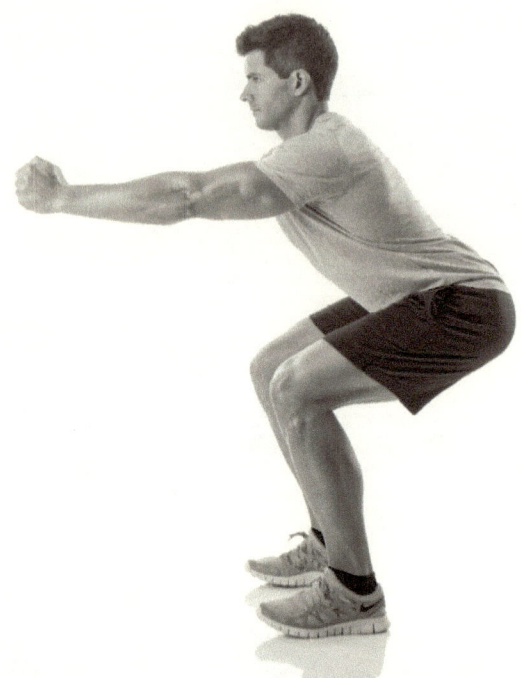

- Stand with legs spread, feet just a little more than shoulder width apart. (Pointing the feet outward slightly helps with balance.)

- Bend your knees and drop your hips to replicate the act of sitting down on a chair.

- Lower yourself so that your thighs are parallel to the ground, then go just a little farther – slightly below parallel.

- Maintain balance with arms stretched out before you and your feet on the floor.

- To return to the starting position, push off through your heels and straighten your legs.

- Try to keep your torso upright, leaning forward only as far as necessary to maintain balance and perform the squat.

Standard Leg Lifts

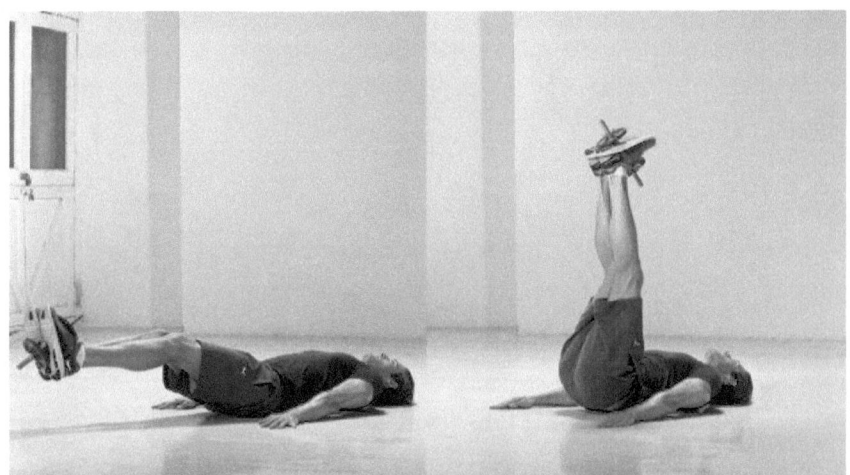

- Lay flat on the floor, with legs extended and hands slightly away from your hips, palms down. (For those with back issues, place a folded towel under your lower back, just above your hips or place hands under your butt.)

- One option is to bend your legs so that your thighs are straight up and your shins are parallel to the floor.

- You then straighten your legs, slowly lowering your feet to about 1 inch above the floor for 1 rep before bringing your knees back up.

- The second option is to bend your legs, then extend them while pointing your toes to the ceiling before lowering the straight legs to just over the floor.

- Another option is to lift your legs straight up off the floor without bending the knees and then lowering them, still straight.

- Repeat for a total of 5 reps in a set. Avoid arching the back by holding the abs tight, breathing out as you lift your legs, and breathing in as you lower them.

Superman

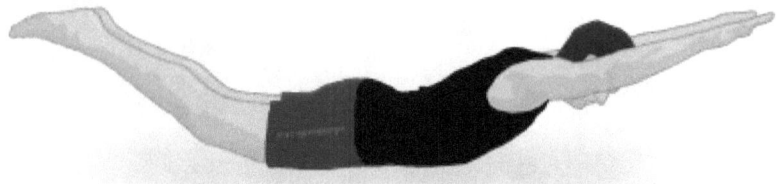

- Lie on your belly, arms straight out in front.
- Lift your arms and legs off the floor without locking joints.
- The goal is to create an arch with shoulders and hips off the floor.
- Hold for 3 to 5 seconds and return to the start.

12 ADDITIONAL CALISTHENICS AND BODYWEIGHT EXERCISES

Arm Circles

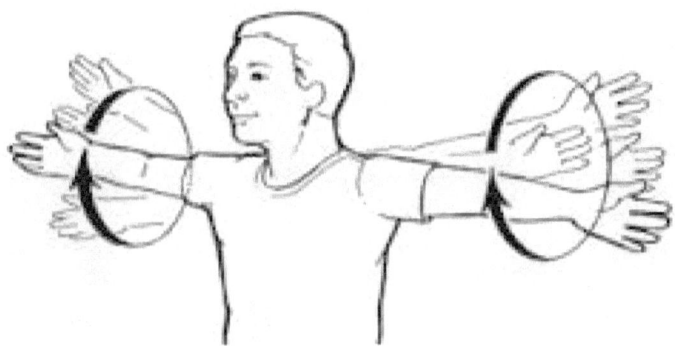

- Standing with feet shoulder width apart (or sitting upright), stretch your arms full length to the sides at shoulder height.

- Perform small circular motions forward for 15 to 20 reps.

- Reverse the circle and continue for another 15 to 20 reps.

- In different sets, vary the size or speed of the circles to work different muscles.

Bend and Reach

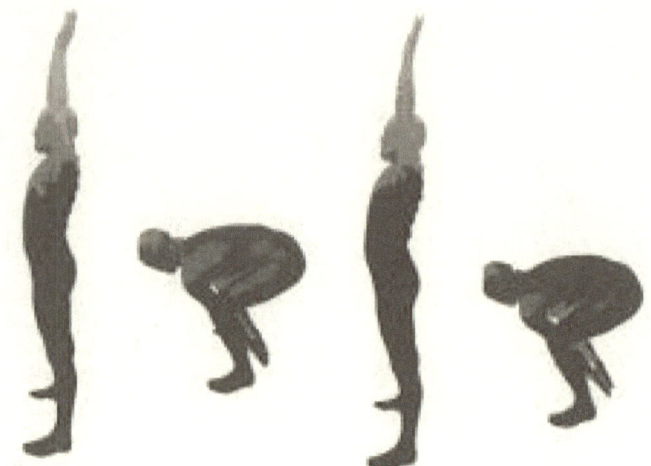

- Begin in a standing position, feet just beyond shoulder width and arms extended so your hands are above your head.

- Squat, keeping your feet full against the floor and your arms extended.

- Round your back as you squat and reach back between your legs as far as possible.

- Return to the standing position for 1 complete rep.

Calf Raises

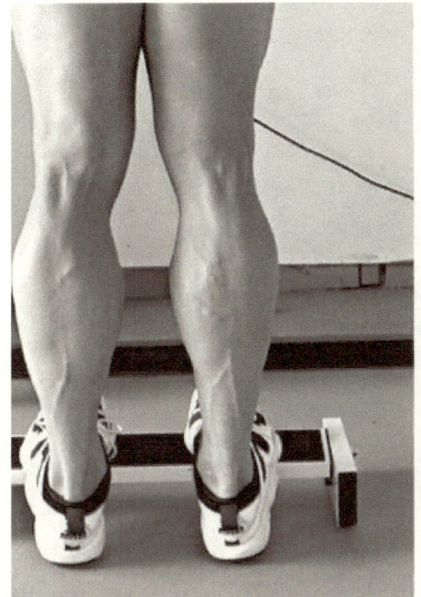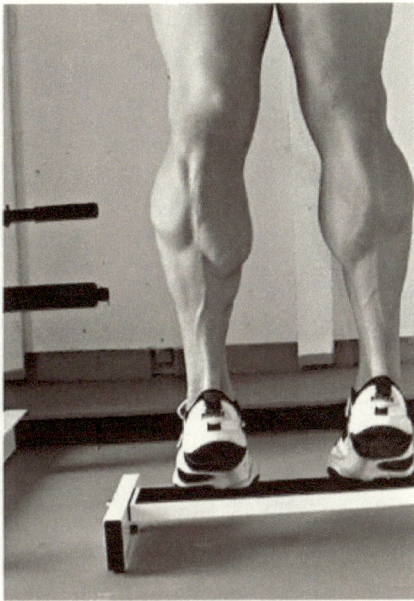

- Stand with your feet close together. Support yourself with your hands if needed.

- Raise up on your toes and hold for 5 seconds.

- Lower your heel to the floor slowly using control.

- For variety, work on one foot at a time or stand on a step or secure platform so your heels can sink below the level of your toes.

Dips

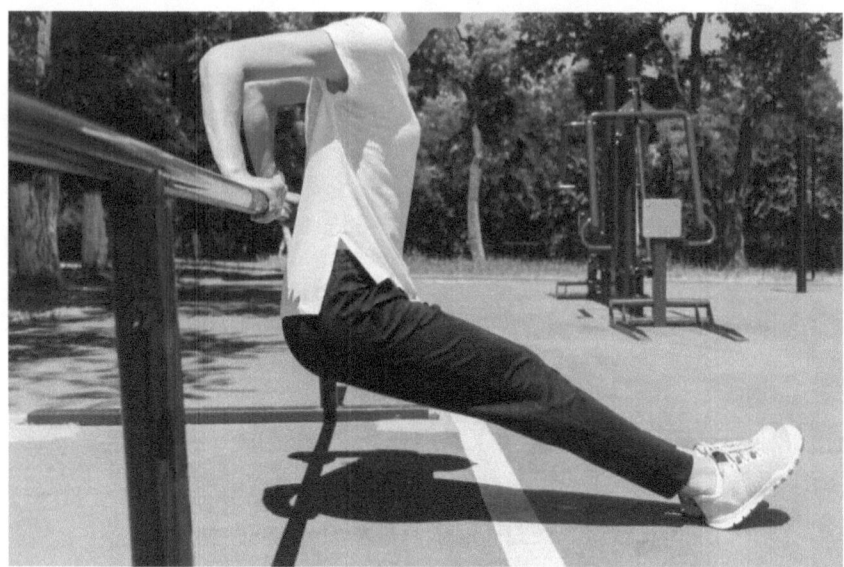

- Stand with your back to a sturdy bench, platform, or low bar. Stretch your legs out to the front while holding the edge with your hands.

- Lean forward slightly and lower your body, bending at the elbows, until your elbow reaches about a 90-degree angle.

- Raise yourself up to a full arm extension using your triceps muscles.

Free Hand Neck Resistance – Front, Back, and Sides

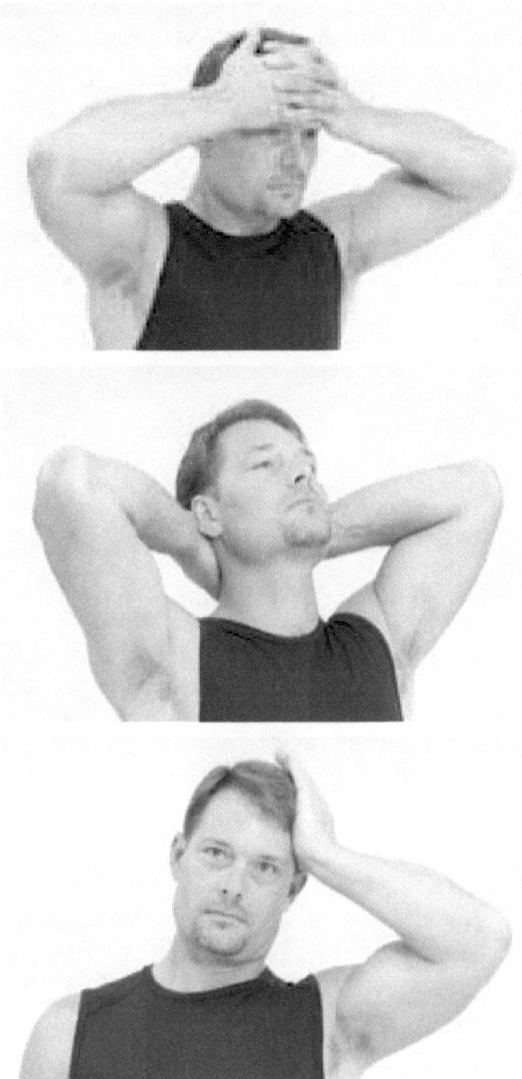

- Stand comfortably, feet shoulder width apart.
- (Front) With your fingers interlocked and hands against your forehead, press your head against your hands.
- Start with your head back and push into your hands, which are providing resistance.
- (Back) Again with fingers interlocked, place your hands on the back of the head.

93

- Starting with your head forward, press back, against your hands.
- (Side) Place your palm against the side of your head and provide resistance as you push your head to that side.
- Switch to work the opposite side.

Mountain Climbers

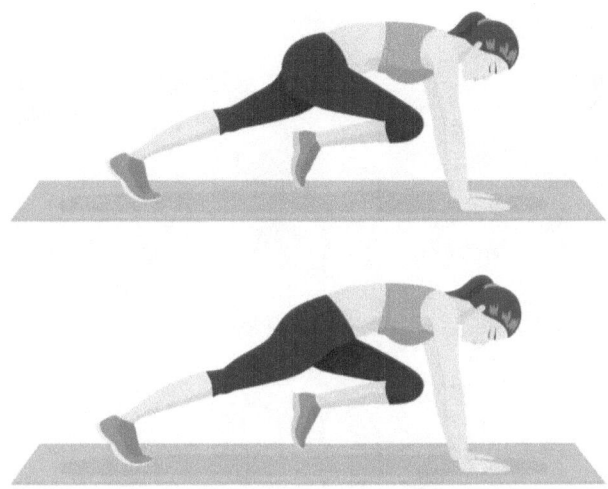

- Begin by kneeling, put your palms on the floor at shoulder width.
- Raise up on your toes and jump to bring one leg up under your chest and the other extended out behind you.
- Jump again to switch so that your legs are in the opposite position for 1 complete rep.
- Maintain a steady pace and hold your core muscles tight.

Neck Rolls

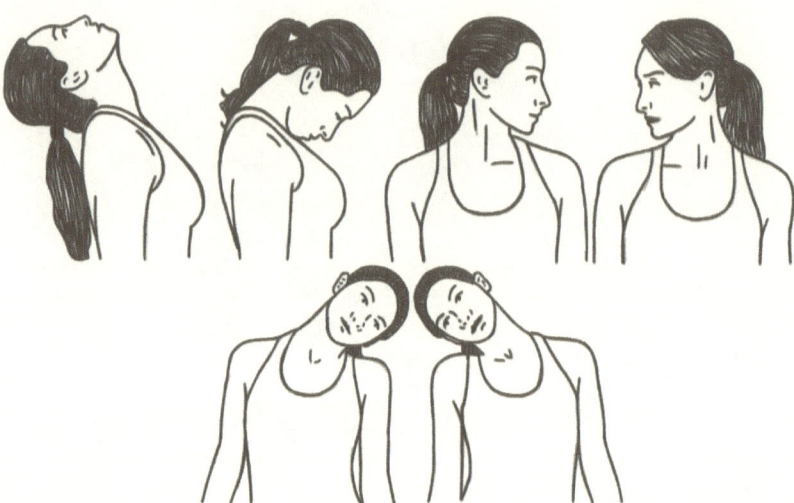

- Standing or sitting upright, bend your head forward bringing your chin towards your chest.
- Roll your head to the right, trying to touch your ear to the right shoulder.
- Roll your head to the back and lift your chin as high as possible.
- Roll your head to the left, trying to touch your ear to the left shoulder.
- Complete two full rotations, rest for 30 seconds, then repeat in the counter-clockwise direction (to the left).

Prisoner Squats

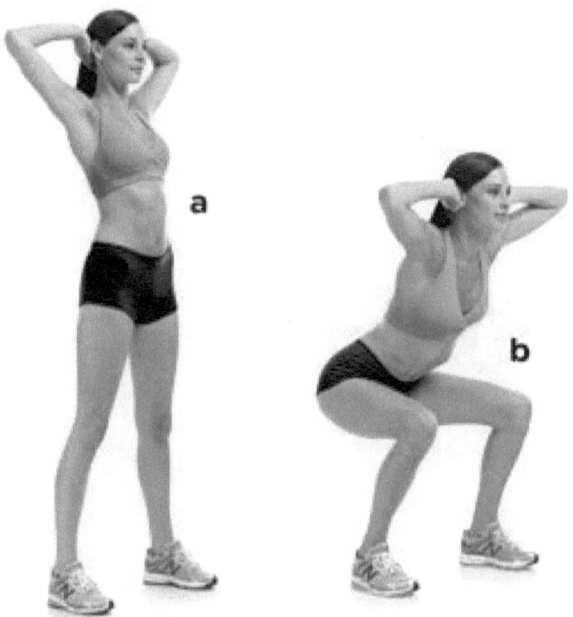

- Stand up straight, legs shoulder width apart, hands behind your head. Elbows and shoulders should be back and your core braced.

- Lower your hips down and back as you bend your knees.

- Drop your hips and bend your knees in 90-degree angles. Press your feet against the floor to support your weight and the downward movement.

- Hold for a few seconds and slowly raise yourself back up using your thighs and hips.

Russian Twists

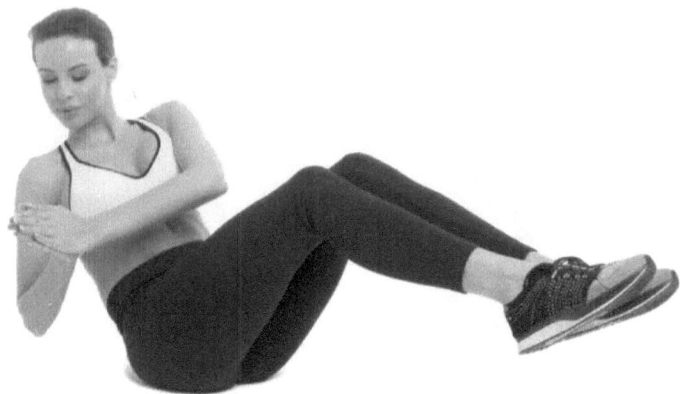

- Sitting on the ground, bend your knees and press your feet together.

- Form a V with your body, bringing your bent knees in toward your chest without touching, then turn your shoulders slowly from side to side, twisting from the waist.

- The further you hold your hands from your body, the harder it will be! Begin with your hands crossed over your chest, then extended in front with your elbows tight to your sides. Finally, loosely hold them out in front of you.

- The slower you twist, the more core tightening you will achieve.

- Raise your feet off the floor for a more intense workout.

Step-Ups

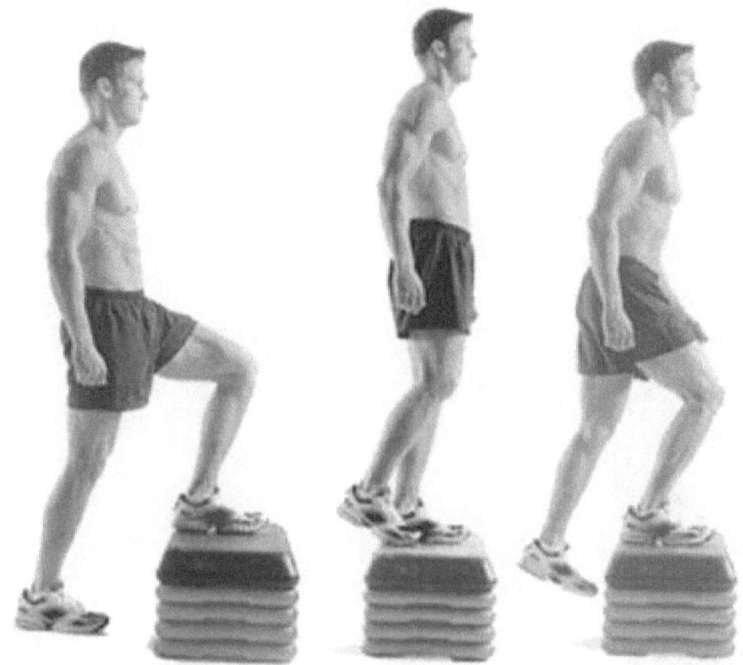

- This is just like climbing up steps, but you are only using one.
- Standing up straight, step up onto a step or sturdy platform.
- After fully straightening the leg, return your other foot to the floor.
- Complete your reps with one leg, then switch to the other side.

Straight Leg (Romanian) Deadlift

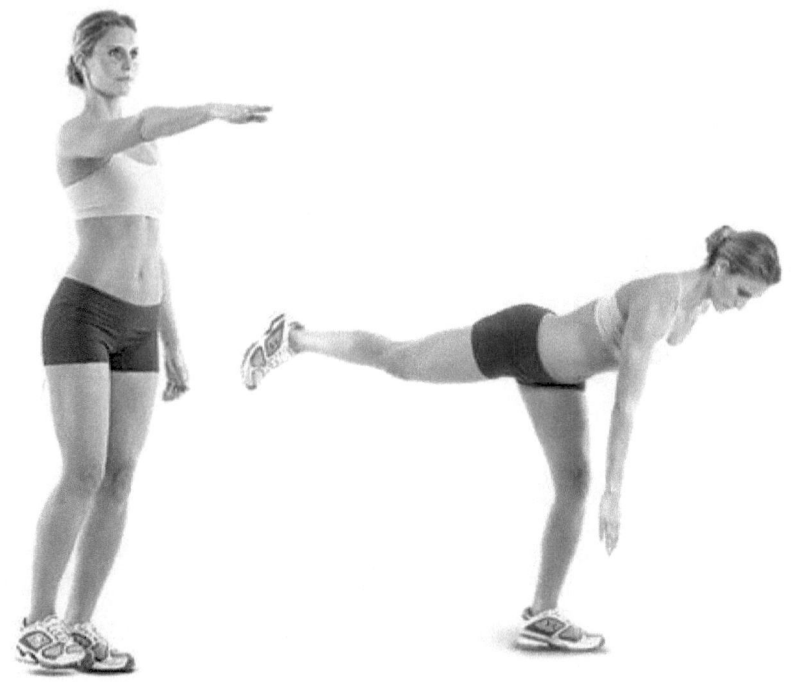

- Stand with feet slightly separated.
- As you bend from the hips with a straight back, lift your right leg up behind you.
- Bend your left knee slightly for balance and bring your torso and leg parallel to the floor.
- Return to the standing position and switch legs for 1 full rep.

The Windmill

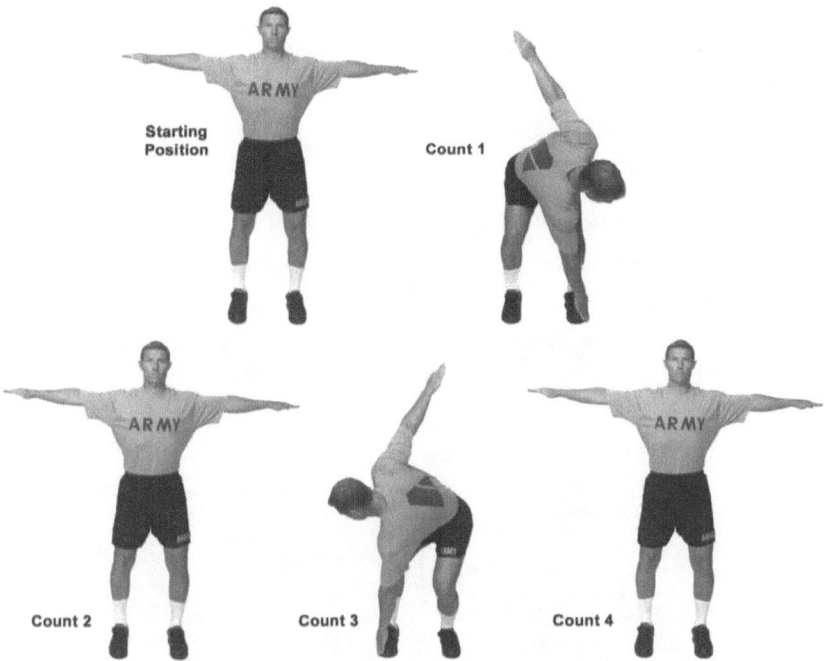

- Standing with feet just beyond shoulder width, extend your arms out from the shoulders, palms facing down.

- Begin rotating to the left from the waist keeping arms in a straight line and head in line with the spine (not bent or turned).

- Bend at the hips and bend knees slightly as you reach down and touch your foot with your fingertips.

- Bring yourself back to the standing position. Perform the stretch to the opposite side for 1 complete rep.

A SPECIAL NOTE ABOUT THE HANDSTAND

Handstands are not necessarily considered to be exercises, but since progressing to handstand push-ups is part of the overall Cals and BWT plan, it deserves to be mentioned.

To simply get the feel for holding your body upright over your head, it may be easiest to **start with a headstand**:

- Get down into a push-up position on your knees.
- Place your head on the floor between your hands with your elbows at 90 degrees.
- Lift your bottom up and balance your weight on your head and hands.
- Place your knees on your elbows for support, then lift your legs, one at a time, up into the air.

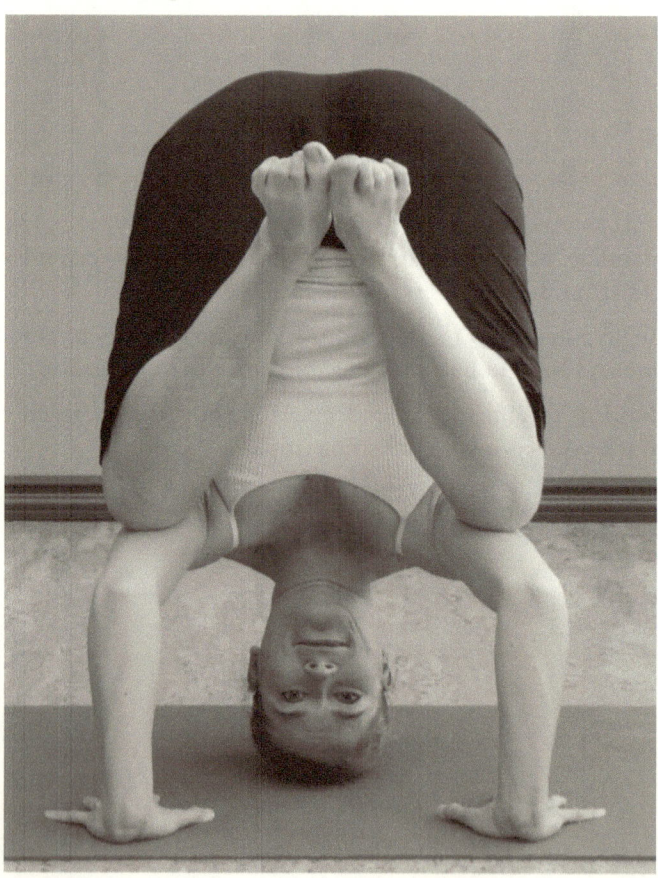

Once you get a feel for the balance, try for the **handstand**. This may require a spotter to help you raise your feet up and to support you as you try to establish stability.

- Lean forward as if you were doing a one-legged dead lift.

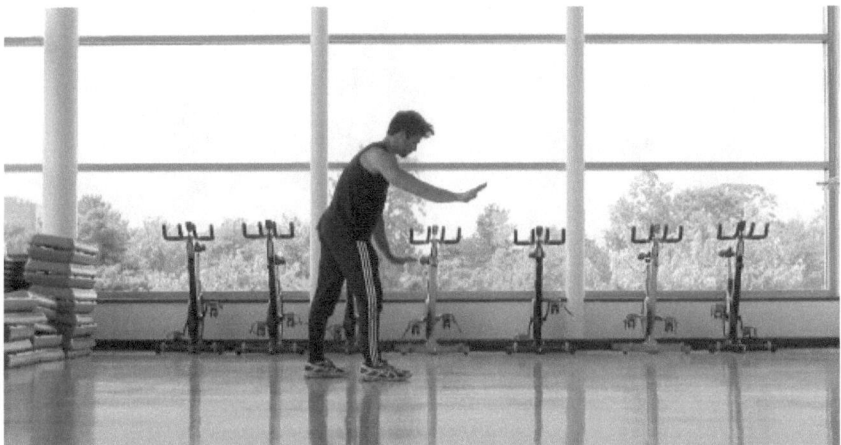

- As you reach for the ground with your hands, push off with the foot on the ground

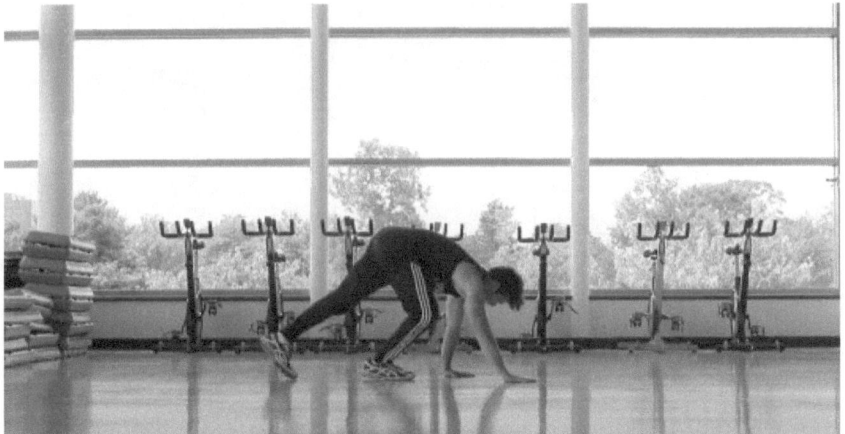

- Bring both feet up together and flex your hands to try to achieve balance

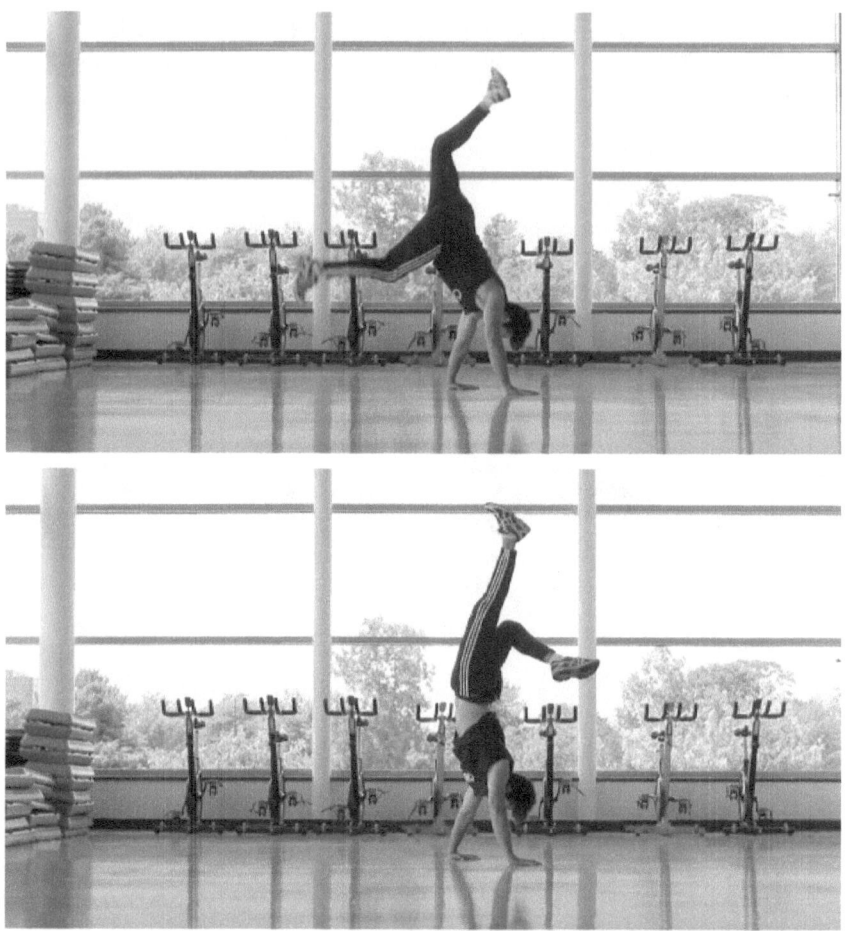

This will probably require quite a few attempts as you get the feel of up-ending yourself. This is the part where muscle control and the intentional maneuvering of your body through space play a huge role!

Another option for learning to perform a handstand involves using a prop, such as a wall or tree.

- From a shortened push-up position, press your feet against the prop.

- 'Walk' your feet up the prop as you walk your hands closer to it.

- When you are relatively upright, try to remove both feet from the support and develop your balance.

- Once you have the strength and balance to hold the handstand, try to get into the position from the upright, free-standing position as instructed above.

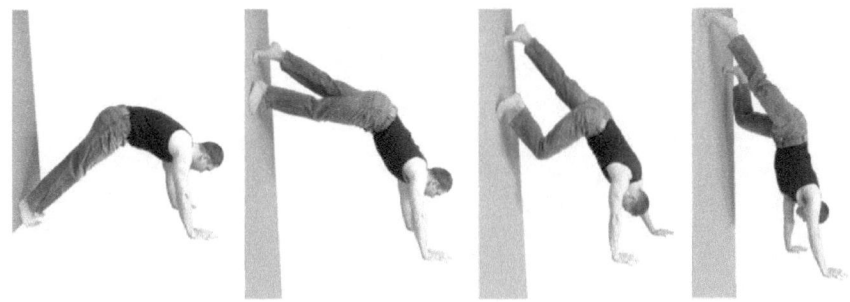

CHAPTER 8

Calisthenics And Bodyweight Training Programs

There is no excuse for anyone to stay out of shape. The simplicity of calisthenics and bodyweight training exercises make a program possible for people of all ages, shapes, and physical conditions. With so many possible exercises and countless variations, beginners and professional athletes as well as disabled and rehabbing people can benefit from Cals and BWT for strength, endurance, and flexibility.

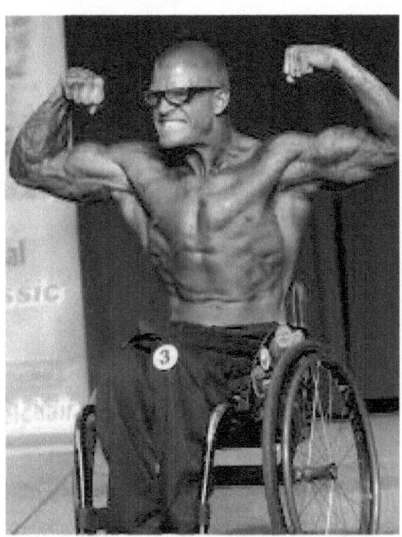

For people accustomed to physical fitness activities, it is not difficult to work calisthenics and bodyweight training into any existing program. The beauty is that the results of this type of workout are so remarkable you will make it your primary means of training!

People who are just getting started should always consult with their healthcare professional to gauge how much to do and how quickly to progress. No matter your condition, though, there are plenty of activities to get you moving to build up your stamina and ability to do more.

WARMING UP TO GET STARTED

To reduce the risk of injury, everyone **needs** to perform some warm-up activities before exerting themselves during an exercise program. A few minutes of cardio and some dynamic stretches can make a big difference in the effectiveness of your workout. **The body responds** instinctively to this practice:

- *Cardiovascular responses*: Blood flow is targeted to working muscles and heart rate; stroke volume and systolic blood pressure increase.

- *Circulatory responses*: The increased blood flow enables your cells to remove wastes more easily and is also providing more fluid to the joints for better cushioning.

- *Respiratory responses*: Respiratory muscles are geared up for increased ventilation rate and volume to improve the exchange of gases in the lungs and body tissues.

- *Musculoskeletal responses*: Body temperature rises due to increased blood flow. This helps reduce muscle stiffness and improves range of motion.

- *Nervous system responses*: Neural pathways (the firing of the nerves from the brain to the muscles and back again) are stimulated so that movement patterns occur smoothly.

- *Metabolic responses*: Hormone levels, particularly glucagon, prepare to raise the level of glucose in the blood for greater energy.

Keeping the idea of CNS training in mind, **warm-ups should imitate the movements you intend to perform** in your workout. It is just like reading through a speech before you give it so it flows smoothly and doesn't present any surprises. It also allows you to gently push your range of motion to prepare for the demands of your upcoming routine or athletic event.

Given the importance of warming up, it is important to do it right. These moves are to be done correctly, just like using the proper posture and position for any activity, and not rushed or abbreviated. For simple workouts, 2 to 3 minutes of warm-ups should be enough as long as you are preparing the muscle groups that will be used in your target exercises. More demanding or advanced workouts require up to 5 to 10 minutes of preparatory warm-ups to ensure full-body activation.

When considering warm-up stretches, keep all parts of your body in mind. The first list is comprised of **basic stretches** and the second (much shorter) list includes actual exercises from Chapter 7.

Arms

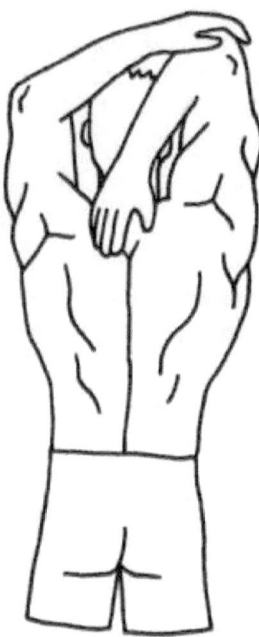

- Stand up straight with your feet at shoulder width.
- Bending your right elbow, send your right hand behind your head.
- Grasp the elbow with the left hand and gently pull, leaning slightly to the left.
- Count to 20, then release. Repeat 2 or 3 times and then switch sides.

Arms and Shoulders

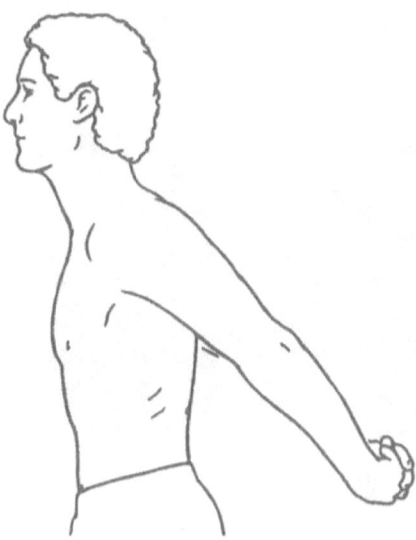

- Stand with your feet at shoulder width.

- Extend arms out behind your back, elbows straight and palms facing one another (link fingers if possible).

- Slightly raise arms up and count to 20, then release. Complete 3 reps.

Arms and Mid Back

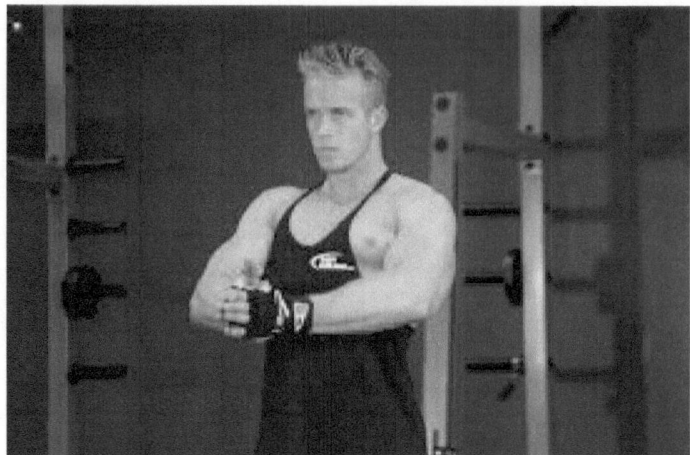

- Stand with feet at shoulder width.
- Stretch your arms in front of you, elbows straight and palms facing one another (link fingers if possible).
- Without leaning, push your hands forward.
- Hold this stretch for a count of 20, then release. Complete 3 reps.

Back, Core, and Obliques

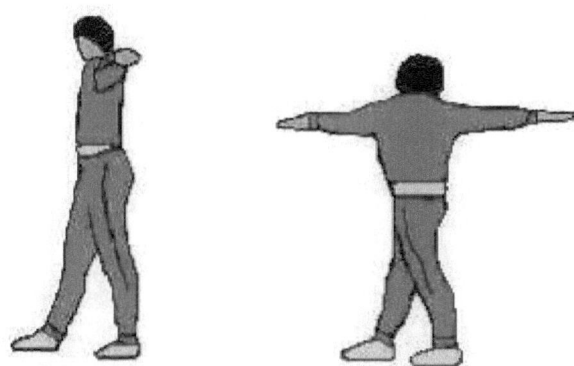

- Stand straight with feet just beyond shoulder width. Extend arms at shoulder height.

- Gently twist your upper body as far as you can to one side without leaning forward.

- Hold for 20 to 30 seconds and return to a forward-facing position.

- Repeat 2 or 3 times and switch sides (or alternate sides for a total of 4 to 6 twists).

Calf and Quad Stretch

- Stand with feet slightly spread, about two feet apart, and facing a wall.

- With heels flat on the floor and maintaining a straight back, lean forward toward the wall.

- Hold for 15 to 20 seconds, relax, and repeat 2 or 3 times.

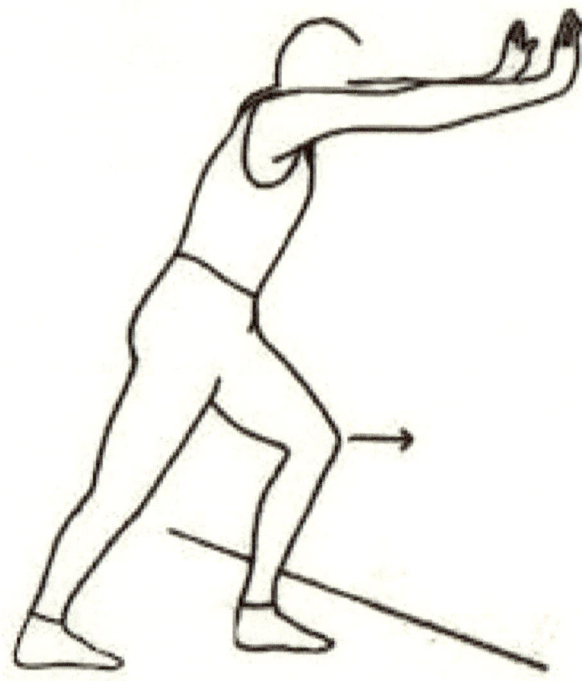

- Then, supporting yourself with your right hand against the wall, raise your right foot and grasp it behind you with your left hand.

- Gently pull your foot back towards your butt, holding for 20 to 30 seconds, then relax.

- Repeat 2 or 3 times and switch sides.

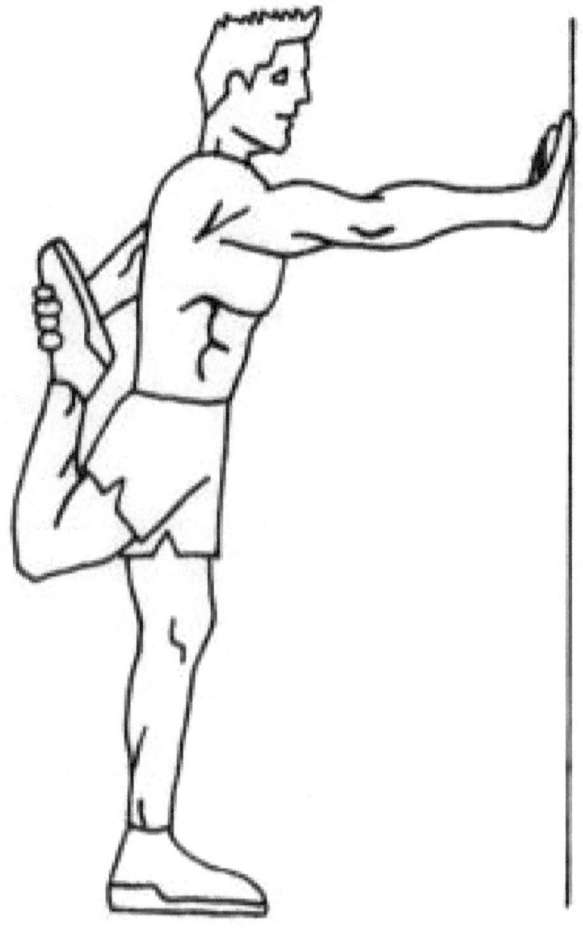

Legs

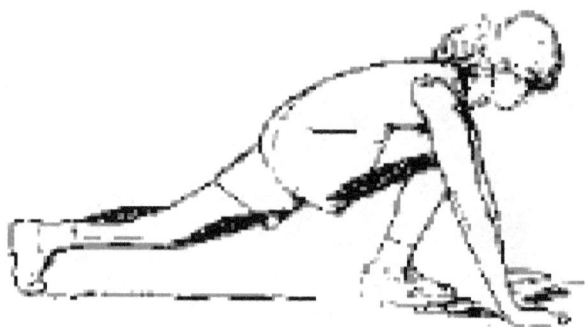

- Squat and place both hands on the floor between your legs.
- Stretch one leg out straight behind you, keeping the other foot flat on the floor.
- Lean forward over your bent knee, holding for 20 to 30 seconds.
- Shift your weight to the back, extended leg and hold for 20 to 30 seconds.
- Relax and repeat for 2 or 3 stretches and switch legs.

Hamstrings

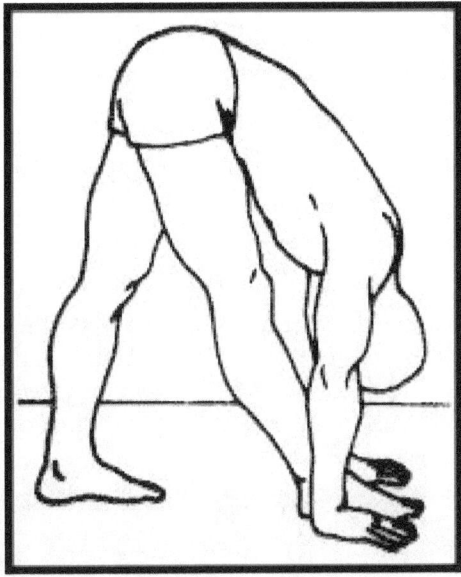

Note that there are many options for stretching the hamstrings, and this is just one!

- Stand up straight with one foot a good foot-step length ahead.

- Bend from the waist, keep your back straight, and reach for the floor on either side of your toes.

- Hold for 20 to 30 seconds, relax, and repeat 2 or 3 times, then switch sides.

EXERCISES THAT DOUBLE AS WARM-UP STRETCHES

- *Arms* – forearms, biceps, and triceps – Arm Circles, Push-Ups

- *Back* – upper, mid, and lower – Superman, Bend and Reach

- *Hips, abs, and obliques* – Planks, Windmill

- *Legs* – calf, thigh, quad, hamstring, groin, ankle – Step-Ups, Calf Raises

- *Neck and shoulders (traps)* – Neck Roll, Free Hand Neck Resistance

Equally as important as the warm-up, the **cool down** offers the body a chance to purge cellular wastes and lactic acid that build up during exercise. Similar stretches as those for the warm-up and slow walking help to bring respiration back to normal and prevent the occurrence of muscle cramps by releasing the tension caused by intense contraction.

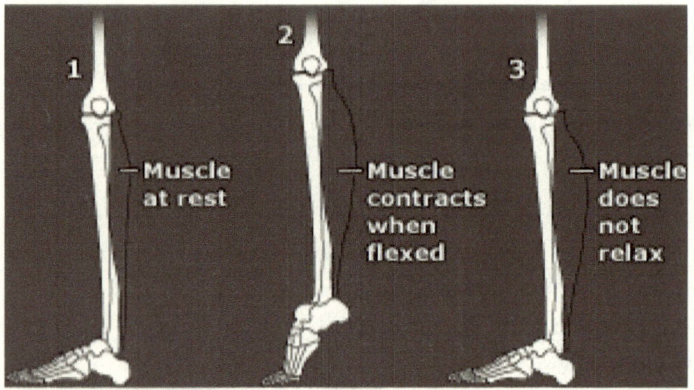

If you ever feel that you have to skip warm-ups or cool downs, **skip or shorten the warm-up**. Since you warm up to prevent muscle strain, it is not something you have to worry about as much with Cals and BWT as you would with weight lifting or other types of intense strength workouts. You can do simpler variations of Cals and BWT exercises as part of the workout and build up intensity, but you *always* have to give your body an opportunity to return to 'normal' after any type of activity.

BEGINNER LEVEL WORKOUT PLAN

The most basic workout plan involves **the 5 major exercises** (and don't forget warm-ups and cool downs!):

1. Dips
2. Lunges
3. Pull ups
4. Push ups
5. Squats

Based on your fitness level, begin with a set number of each of these exercises, such as 5 or 8. If that is too easy, begin with 10 and/or **add a few additional items**, such as:

- Crunches
- The Windmill
- Calf Raises

Gradually add 1 or 2 reps each week until you double your starting number of reps. Drop back to that starting number again but do 2 full sets, building up the number of reps each week. Take a short rest break (1 or 2 minutes) between sets to catch your breath but not long enough to cool down. As you work comfortably with the number of reps in each set, cut back on the rest in between.

Once you are able to do 3 sets comfortably, drop down the number of reps halfway to your original starting number and **add one exercise at a time** from the list in Chapter 7, such as:

- Burpees
- Russian Twists
- Bridges
- Superman
- Leg Lifts
- Mountain Climbers
- Step-ups
- Prisoner Squats

Be sure to select a variety of motions that target different muscle groups for a full-body workout. Remember to maintain proper form and a tight core. Do not increase your reps if your technique suffers! It is better to do a few exercises correctly than a lot of them wrong – you could be preventing true progress or even be heading for injury!

A WORD ABOUT TIMING

Timing your workouts is an important part of balancing your results. For beginners, performing calisthenics and bodyweight exercises 2 or 3 times a week for 20 to 30 minutes is a good goal. It also depends on the types of exercises you include in your workout. It has already been stated that you have to choose exercises that **hit different muscle groups**. Another consideration is **balancing cardio and strength** as well as impact and non-impact choices to prevent strain on the joints and muscles.

Swimming is an excellent option that is very gentle on the joints. Many of the Cals and BWT can be done in the water, which protects the joints and offers support while providing added resistance. Older people and those in need of physical therapy can reap great benefits by exercising in the water, and it is also a terrific break for any athlete who needs to tone it down a little.

Once you are in a steady routine and are progressing with your endurance and strength, it is possible to increase your workouts to 4, 5, or even 7 a week. Just keep balance in mind, alternating days of predominantly cardio with days of primarily strength exercises. (You can actually do many of the same exercises for both purposes – quickly for cardio and more slowly for strength!)

Another surprising option is to perform some type of activity that increases your heart rate in several shorter periods as long as you achieve a total of 30-60 minutes in a day. This is perfect for busy people because you can climb stairs instead of using an elevator, rake leaves or mop a floor, carry a child, bag of groceries, or a laundry basket – you get the idea! Not only can you get a full workout in, you double the metabolic boost you get and increase afterburn by firing it up more than just once.

LEAVE TIME FOR REST

While simple calisthenics and bodyweight exercises may be done every day, it is important to recognize the body's need for rest. This is especially true when you are involved in more complex, higher intensity workouts that last until you experience 'the wall' or muscle failure. The muscles grow in mass and increase in strength by being broken down and then rebuilding. This rebuilding must have a chance to take place, so **strength training workouts should have 24-48 hour breaks** for those specific muscle groups.

To be more specific, pull-ups, dips, and squats require a large degree of strength and wider muscle recruitment, particularly when you are doing large numbers of reps and sets. They should not be done every day in order to allow those muscles to rest and your cellular energy to be restored. Offset those exercises with more stretches and cardio-based choices on alternate days.

Even endurance training demands some downtime, at least once a week or every 10 days at the most. If you can't simply rest, take a slow walk, doggy-paddle in a pool, or do some basic yoga. This is good for your mind as well as your body.

In addition to rest from muscular efforts, it is also crucial that you get enough sleep daily. Sleep deprivation accounts for a wide range of negative effects, the most significant of which (in terms of weight management and fitness) include the disruption of hormone secretion (related to diabetes and Human Growth Hormone for muscle repair and building) and also the impact on the quality of food choices we make.

INCREASE YOUR INTENSITY WITH PROGRESSIVE TRAINING

Calisthenics and bodyweight exercises can help anyone build a better body. While Cals and BWT are best suited for endurance and lean muscle mass, **strength and pumped up muscles** can also be **achieved by increasing the intensity** of Cals and BWT workouts.

Different positions of the same exercise target slightly different muscle groups.

- With push-ups and pull-ups, hold the hands closer to mid-line and farther than shoulder width apart to create all around definition and mass.

- Adding leg raises and/or a torso twist to a pull-up leads to killer abs.

- Doing one-armed or one-legged push-ups, squats, and other exercises doubles the intensity.

- Demanding greater balance causes more muscles to become involved.

Developing complete control over your muscles and their function is what creates a powerful body. Again, picture a gymnast performing a routine, a ballet dancer or a martial arts expert: total concentration and a highly developed CNS connection between the brain and muscles allows for moves that all but defy gravity. This occurs only after tremendous amounts of repetition and long hours of practice, during which the difficulty of the exercise is steadily increased. Initially, reps and sets are needed to increase and develop strength, flexibility, and endurance, but the **real power and muscle-building comes from more difficult fully functional movements** that utilize multiple joints and a variety of stabilizer muscles. This is where Cals and BWT are so different from weight lifting!

This is called '*Progressive Training*,' and it involves only the basic exercises with a large number of progressively more difficult variations. Changing the range of motion and leverage of the body along with overall positioning provides the escalating difficulty. From an on-your-knees push-up, you can ultimately progress to a handstand push-up and even a one-armed handstand push-up!

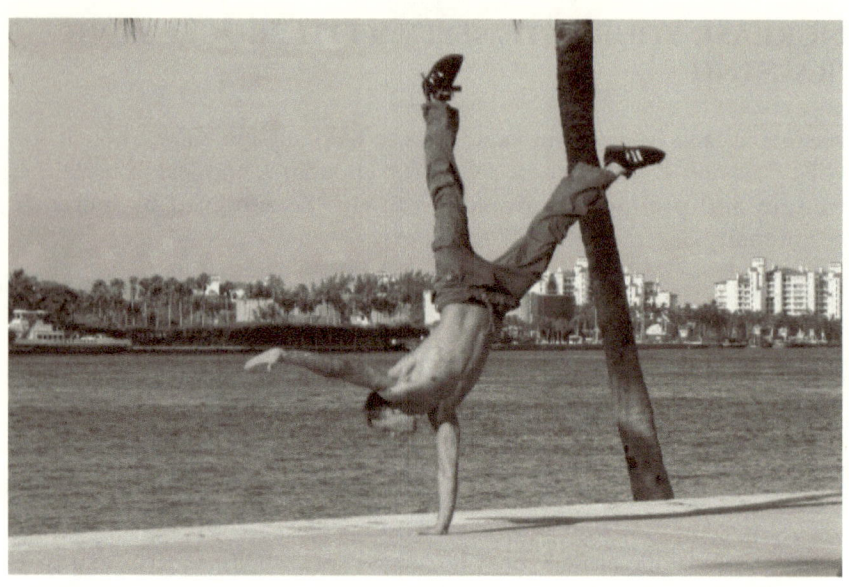

CHAPTER 9

Amping Up The Basic Workout

Anyone can **turn a simple calisthenics and bodyweight training workout into an intense muscle-building session** by applying physics to physiology. What this means is that by making some simple adjustments to your positioning, it is possible to amp up your workout without having to use weights or any other equipment to build muscle and develop a great body.

Just like a child who has to crawl before he can walk, everyone who wants to make great progress using Cals and BWT must start at the beginning. Accuracy of movement and attention to posture and form are key elements in successful muscle building, so mastering the basics is critical to future improvement.

PRINCIPLES OF ADVANCED WORKOUTS

Relatively simple changes in your workout can have a huge impact on your overall results. Looking at some basic facts can add a lot to your program as you master the basics and get ready to move on. This basic understanding of the difference between all-around fitness and weight-lifting principles allows you to reach virtually any goal you set in terms of strength and muscle mass through calisthenics and bodyweight training.

1. **Work harder, not necessarily longer**. The key to building muscle is to perform fewer but more intense reps. Working to exhaustion, taking a rest, and then working the same muscles again in several sets is the key to building muscle.

2. **Isolate key muscles**. While Cals and BWT provide for greater full-body fitness, it is possible to isolate key muscle groups for significant workouts. Focusing on one set of muscles at a time builds those muscles faster.

3. **Divide and conquer**. Following item 2, it is easy to provide rest for a worked muscle group by splitting up your workouts. One day, work on the shoulders and arms, then the next, work on legs. The third day you can focus on the chest and back and then start over the next day with the shoulders and arms. You can train 6 days each week and then take a full day for overall recovery.

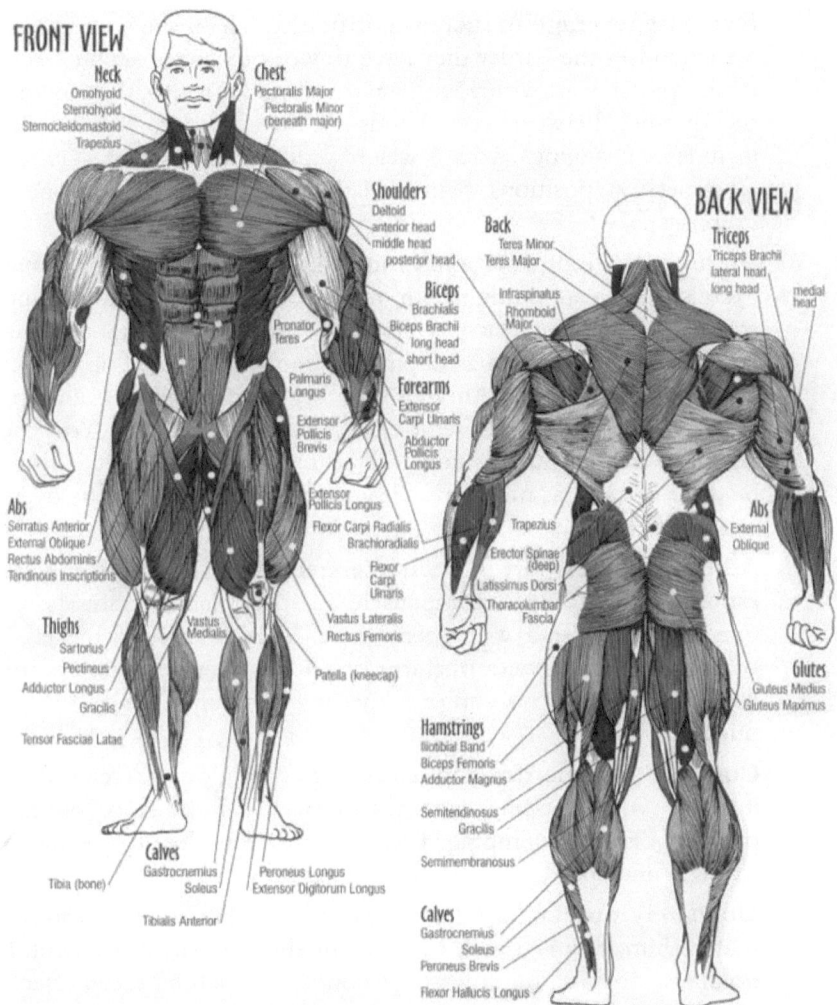

4. **Focus on functional movement.** The beauty of Cals and BWT is that many of the exercises mimic daily activities. Capitalize on that and be sure to include motion in all three planes – side to side, front to back, and rotation or twisting.

5. **Maintain steady, controlled movements.** Bouncing creates a type of momentum, and you don't want that to make the workout easier. Contract the muscles you are working as much as possible and hold the position for at least 5 seconds to increase the time under tension. To force the muscles to work harder, limit rest periods so that lactic acid does not have a chance to dissipate until your training session is complete.

6. **Decrease leverage to increase difficulty**. The more your muscles are extended, the harder they have to work to perform an exercise. Push-ups can start with your hands at shoulder width, then increase the distance between your hands to work harder. This concept includes changing your weight distribution and utilizing asymmetrical positions (which lead up to one-arm and one-leg exercises).

7. **Increase the length of each motion**. This can be done for many exercises such as putting your feet up on a block for push-ups, squats, or lunges; using a higher platform for step-ups, and combining moves such as adding a jump to the stand-up element of simple toe-touches. Another way to get more out of each rep is to begin the move but return only part-way to start. You then return to the full-out position and return normally to start. This can be done once or as mini-reps within each rep to increase the overall work of the muscles.

8. **Add balance as part of each exercise**. By forcing your muscles, especially the core, to compensate for off-balance exercises, you increase the overall work performed. This is easily achieved by performing moves with one arm or one leg or when you progress from a plank to a push-up or a kneeling push-up to an on-the-toes push-up.

9. **Combine plyometrics and isometrics** within one exercise. Add a jump to your stepping exercises or push off the floor during a push-up. Simply jumping fires up the muscles for explosive strength and speed and adds to your cardio workout.

10. **Don't rely on elastic energy**. Muscles are like coiled springs so that each motion is usually followed by the opposite movement. By holding a position for at least 4 seconds, that natural recoil effect is eliminated so the return motion depends completely on the muscle strength.

11. **Aim for progressive overload**. For the greatest improvements in muscle mass, you have to continually demand more from those muscles. Increase sets, the number of times you work out each week, and the difficulty of the exercises you perform (without compromising on good form). 'Convict conditioning,' also referred to as 'old school calisthenics' is a popular plan for progressively increasing the difficulty of exercises to maximize intensity based on the knowledge and techniques from the strongmen, gymnasts, circus performers, and acrobats of old.

12. **Perform supersets to maximize your workout**. A superset involves exercises that target completely different muscle groups so

that you can work each group to near failure, give them a rest, and re-target them for what is called 'density training' and leads to 'cumulative fatigue.' You are performing a low number of reps but many sets within 15 or 20 minutes of work.

ADVANCED CALISTHENICS AND BODYWEIGHT TRAINING EXERCISES

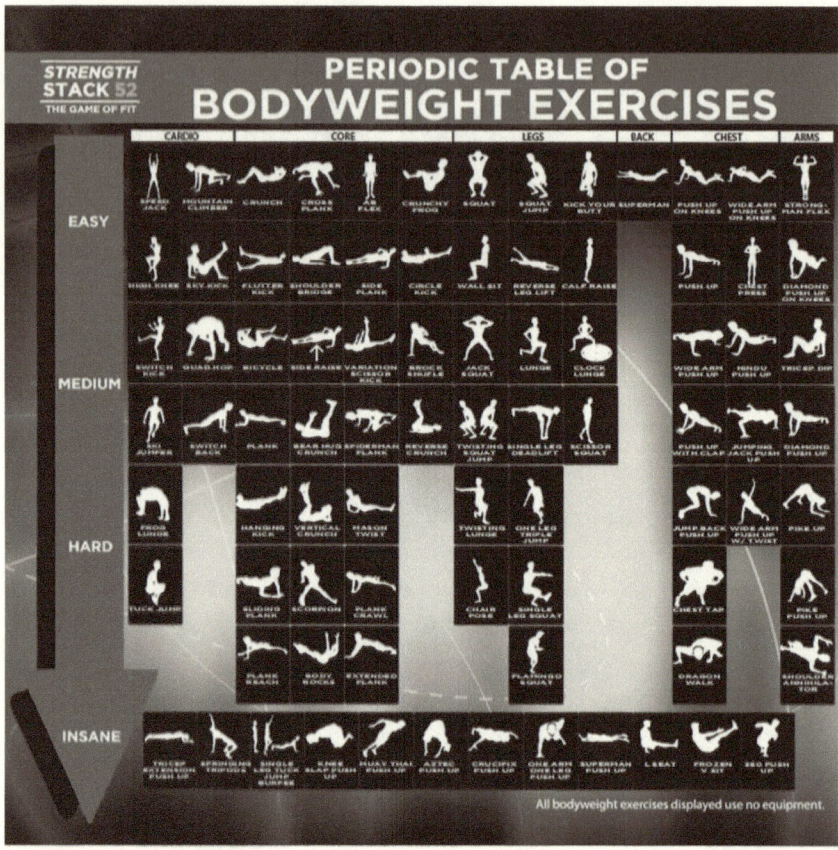

With enough motivation and preparation, everyone can **progress from the basic forms** of calisthenics and bodyweight exercises **to truly amped up versions**. Notice the combined movements utilized in these exercises and how they change weight distribution and length of each motion.

These are highly advanced moves and require plenty of preparation with a wide variety of Cals and bodyweight exercises to build up the necessary strength and agility. You may only be able to perform one or two of these exercises to start, but they will become easier as you follow the steps for improving overall strength and endurance.

One Legged Jumps

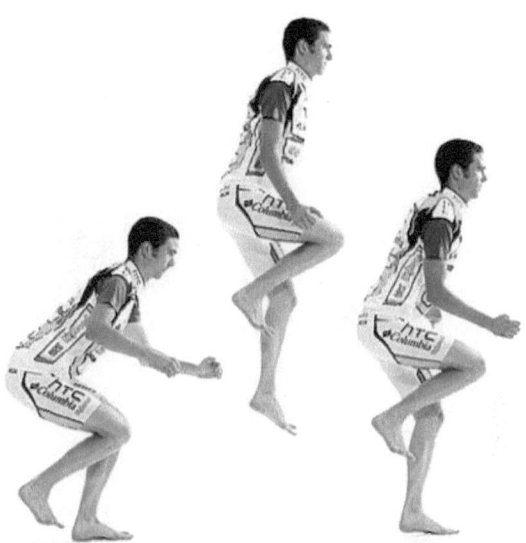

- Balance on one foot and bend that knee slightly to maintain balance.
- While swinging your arms forward, jump off of that foot to the side of the raised foot.
- Continue hopping around the compass points – forward, right, backward, and left – then switch legs.

High Stepping Forward or Reverse Lunge

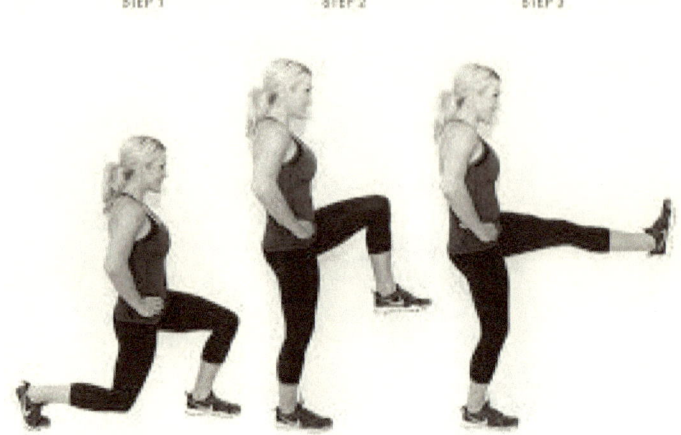

- Stand on one foot and step back with the other into a reverse lunge.

- Push off the back (for forward) or front (for reverse) foot forcefully to stand and bring that knee up to your chest.

- Continue with that foot, placing it in front or behind you in the lunge position, and push off the opposite foot. This should look like exaggerated walking.

Side Lunges

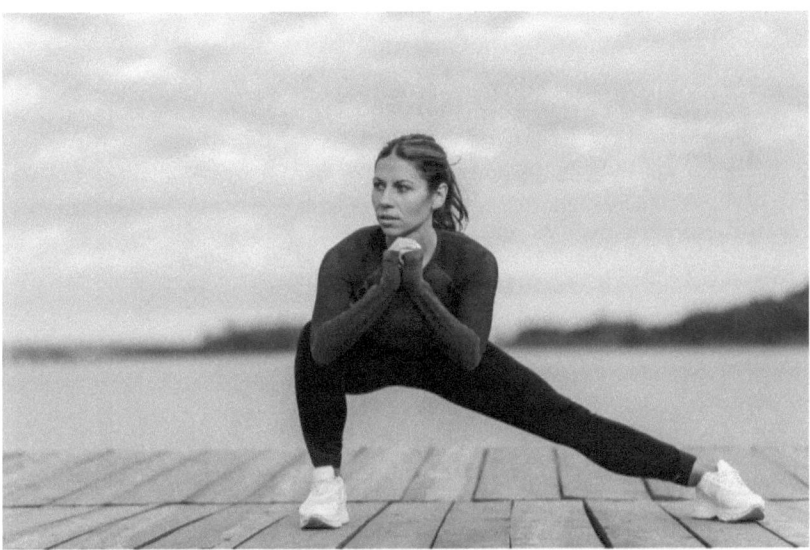

- Stand up straight with feet together.

- Raise your right foot and lunge to the right.

- Keep toes facing forward and your weight on your heels.

- Push off with your right foot and return to the start.

- Alternate sides, pushing explosively to return to the upright position just like a speed skater.

- Make this even more difficult by bending the knee of the extended leg into a side squat.

Plyometric Push-Up

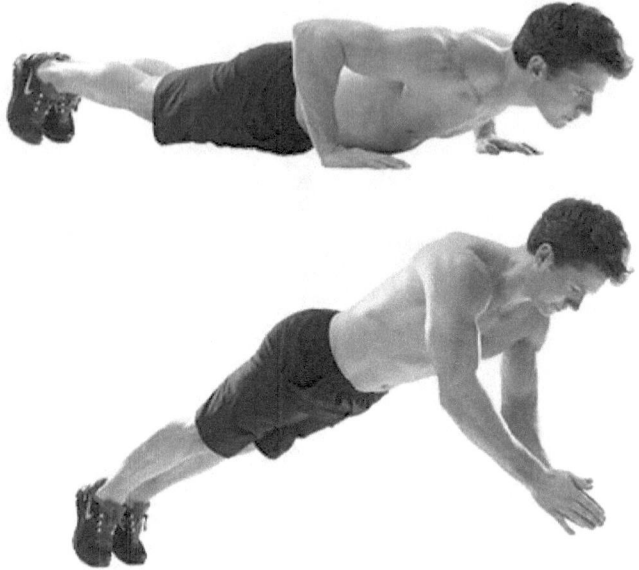

- From a standard push-up position, with elbows close to the body, push up forcefully and clap your hands as you are raised off the ground.

- Begin from your knees and work up to doing them on your toes.

This is a perfect example of an exercise that you may only be able to perform once or twice to start. Continue with regular push-ups and other arm- and shoulder-strengthening exercises as you try to increase your reps with the plyo push-up.

Forward Leaps (Broad Jumps)

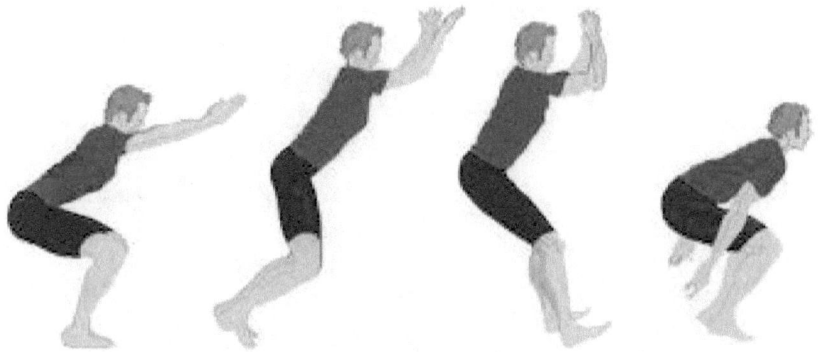

- Stand up straight. Place your feet at hip width.
- Squat while bringing your arms back.
- Spring forward swinging your arms forward and land on the balls of your feet, knees bending slightly to absorb the impact.
- Continue leaping without resting in between.

Hot Foot Tuck Jumps

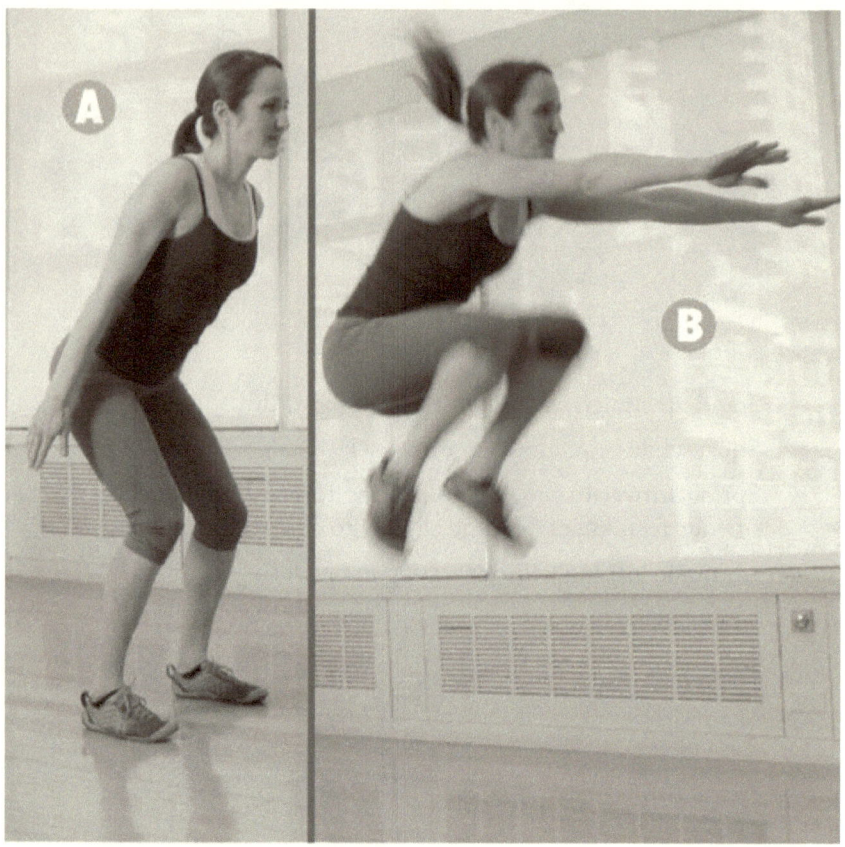

- Starting with feet shoulder width apart, squat down slightly and jump as high as possible.
- Pull your knees up toward your chest.
- Extend your legs and land on your toes.
- Continue into a slight squat and jump up again without resting.

Lunge Jumps

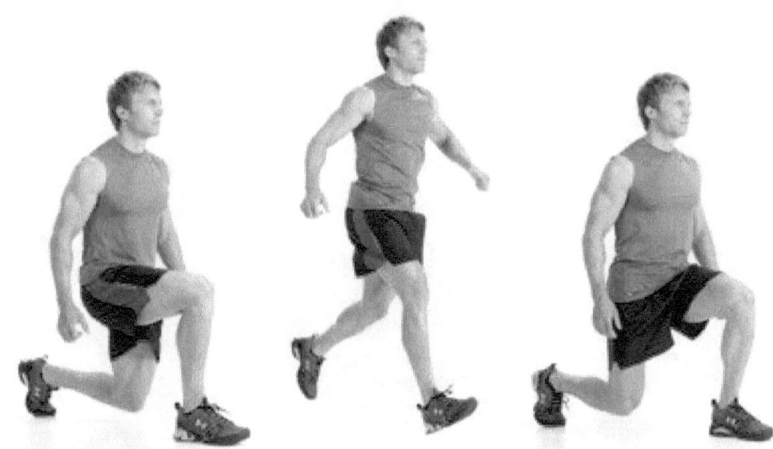

- Stand in a lunge position and jump up as high as possible.
- While in the air, switch legs.
- Without resting, continue jumping, switching legs with each jump.

Star Planks

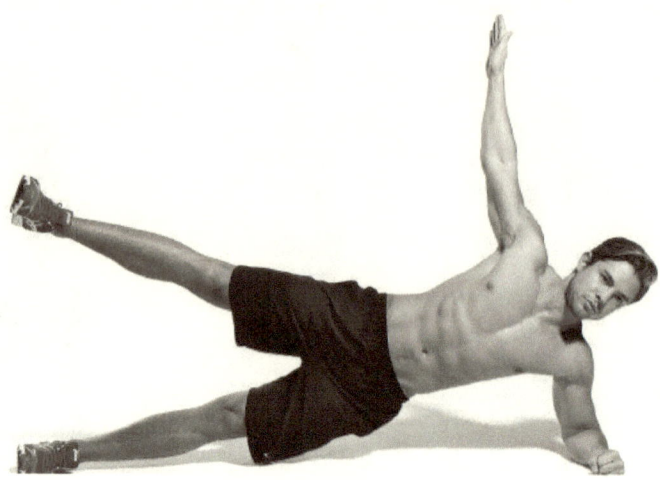

- Begin in a side plank position with your elbow beneath your shoulder.

- Holding your core tightly, lift the top leg with the knee loose as high as possible.

- Hold for 2-3 seconds and lower the leg.

- After several reps, switch sides.

Combo Side and Tuck Jump

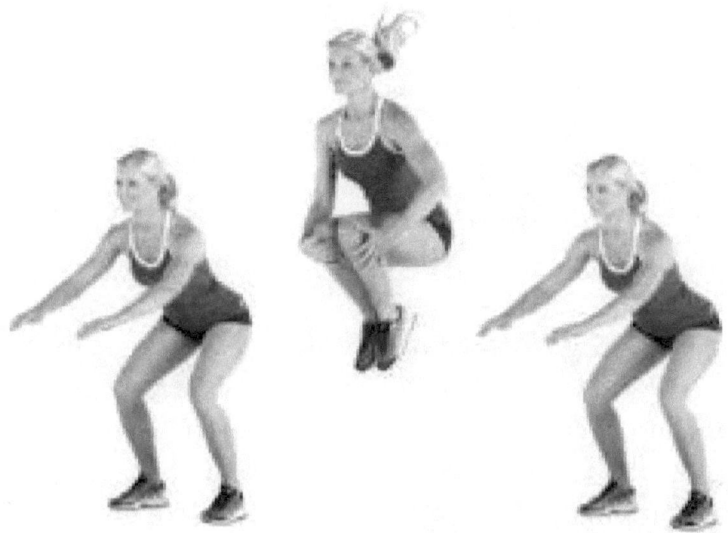

- Stand with your feet together.

- Bend slightly at the knees and jump to the side.

- As soon as you land, bend the knees slightly and perform a tuck jump, lifting your knees up to the chest as high as possible.

- On landing, bend the knees slightly and jump to the opposite side and continue without resting.

Kneeling Squat Jump

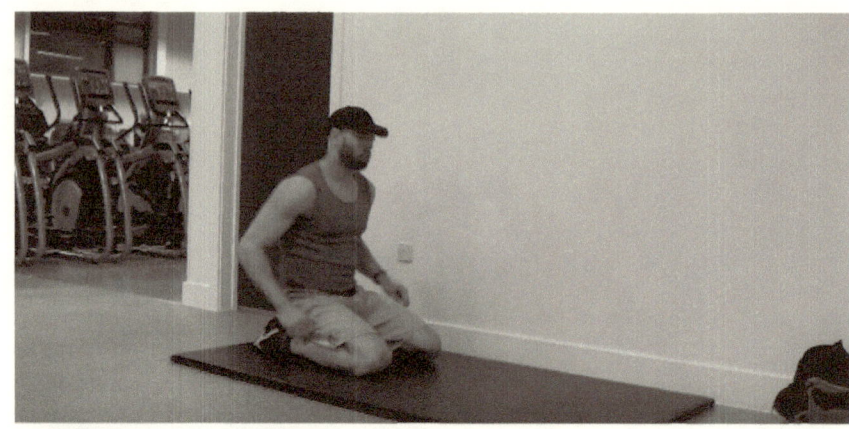

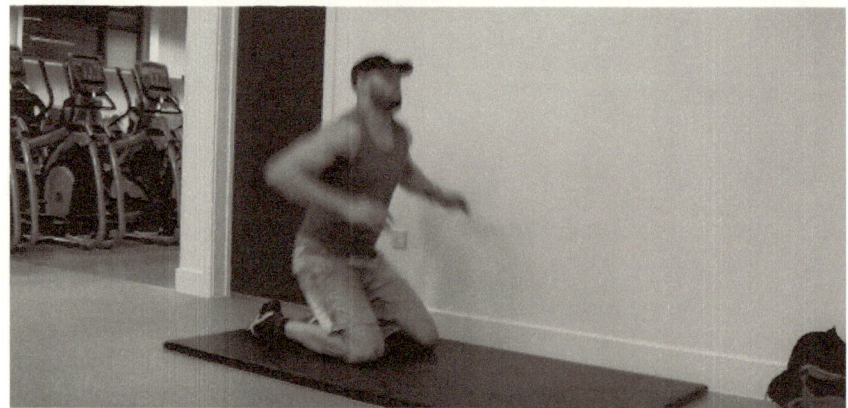

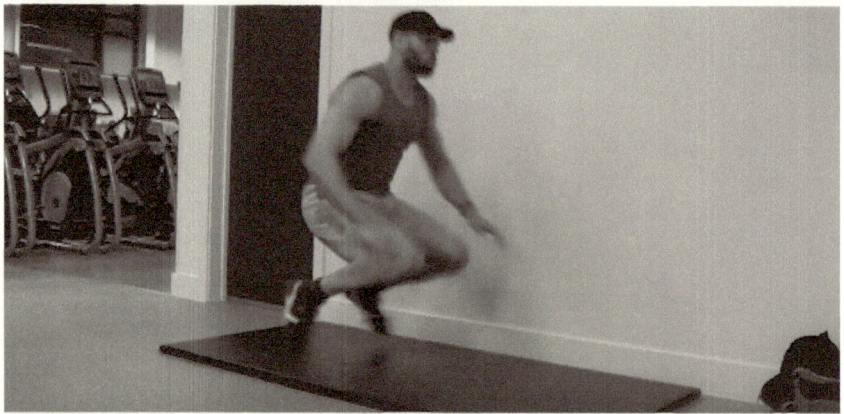

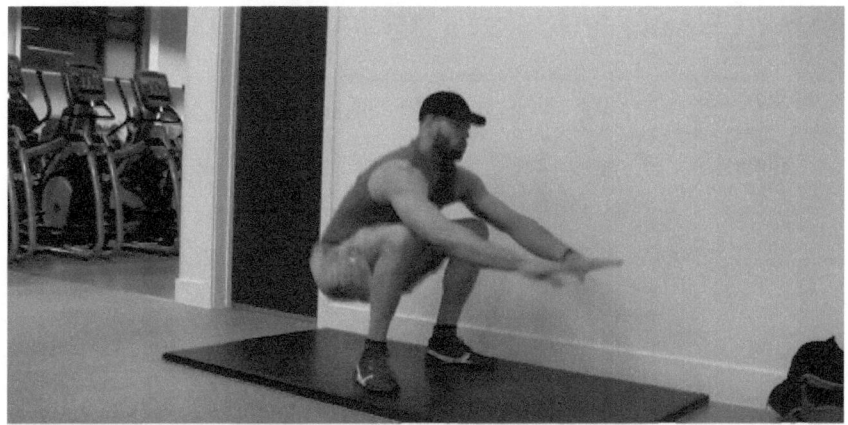

- Begin kneeling with your knees a little wider than your hips.
- Using your arms for force, swing them back, then forward.
- While swinging the arms forward, jump into a squat position.
- Return to the kneeling position and continue.

30-DAY CHALLENGE – 5000 SQUATS & 1000 PUSH-UPS

Day 1	*Day 2*	*Day 3*	*Day 4*	*Day 5*
40 Squats	45 Squats	50 Squats	65 Squats	75 Squats
8 Push Ups	9 Push Ups	10 Push Ups	13 Push Ups	15 Push Ups
Day 6	*Day 7*	*Day 8*	*Day 9*	*Day 10*
85 Squats	90 Squats	100 Squats	115 Squats	125 Squats
17 Push Ups	18 Push Ups	20 Push Ups	23 Push Ups	25 Push Ups
Day 11	*Day 12*	*Day 13*	*Day 14*	*Day 15*
135 Squats	140 Squats	145 Squats	155 Squats	160 Squats
27 Push Ups	28 Push Ups	29 Push Ups	31 Push Ups	32 Push Ups
Day 16	*Day 17*	*Day 18*	*Day 19*	*Day 20*
170 Squats	180 Squats	185 Squats	190 Squats	200 Squats
34 Push Ups	36 Push Ups	37 Push Ups	38 Push Ups	40 Push Ups
Day 21	*Day 22*	*Day 23*	*Day 24*	*Day 25*
210 Squats	220 Squats	230 Squats	240 Squats	250 Squats
42 Push Ups	44 Push Ups	46 Push Ups	48 Push Ups	50 Push Ups
Day 26	*Day 27*	*Day 28*	*Day 29*	*Day 30*
260 Squats	270 Squats	280 Squats	290 Squats	300 Squats
52 Push Ups	54 Push Ups	56 Push Ups	58 Push Ups	60 Push Ups

ABS WORKOUT CHALLENGE

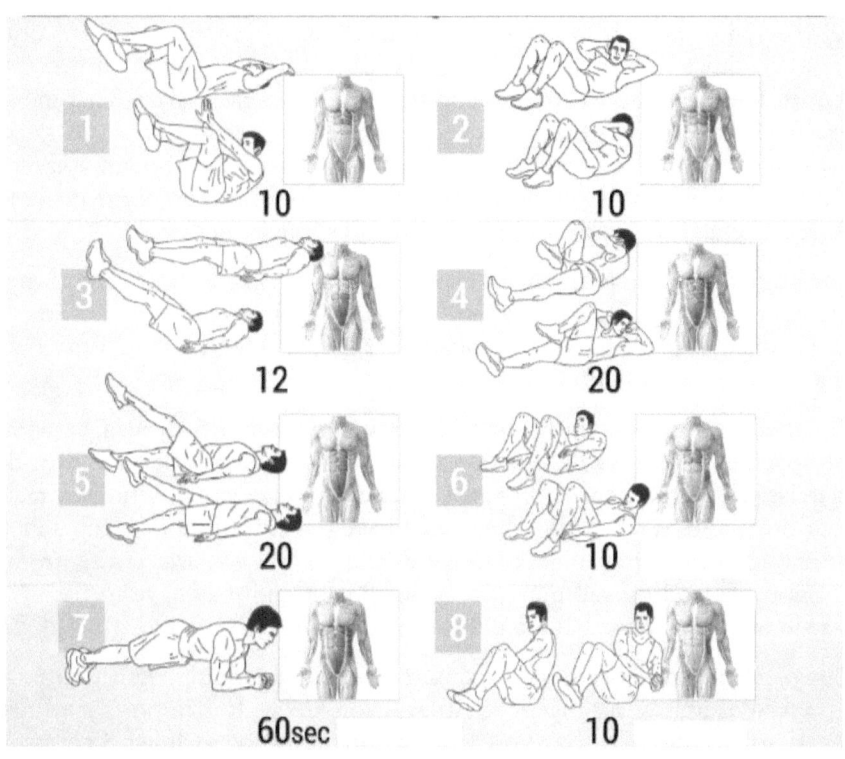

IT WILL TAKE TIME

Although it is possible to quickly see results from 30-minute workouts done 3 or 4 times a week, **patience is** probably **the most important requirement** for successfully adding strength and muscle mass. That means you have to stay focused, stick to a plan, and ignore any excuse to skip a training session. This is particularly true when you feel as though you have hit a plateau. When that happens, mix up the workout – try some different exercises, change your reps and sets, and add some extra cardio.

For beginners, it is fairly easy to see results after only a short time. A new or renewed focus on exercising is usually accompanied with efforts of eating a better diet, and the combination creates a better looking, fitter body in a relatively short period.

For people who already have a good degree of fitness, obvious improvements may take a little longer since you have to not only learn the exercises to perform them properly, you have to give yourself time to reach your optimal reps and sets. You at least have the advantage of being able to work out more since you are in better condition, but you are starting from a position of good overall muscular development and may have to focus on certain muscle groups that are new to the demands of Cals and BWT.

Part of having patience is not assuming you can just jump right into more advanced exercises, no matter what level you are at. It is important to **find the hardest exercise that you can do correctly for at least 5 reps** and then work from there. Since there can be as many as ten steps in the progressive difficulty of some moves and you want to build up to 10-15 reps, everyone will find that there is plenty of room to increase the level of difficulty from their starting workout.

Another aspect of having patience is understanding that not every person is the same. Genetics plays a large role in determining the optimum muscle mass an individual can obtain. That does not mean, however, that you can't create a fit, well-toned, and defined body with plenty of strength. World class weight lifters, body builders, gymnasts, and figure skaters have all achieved peak fitness, but they certainly don't all look alike!

KNOW YOUR BODY TYPE

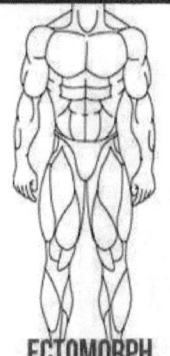
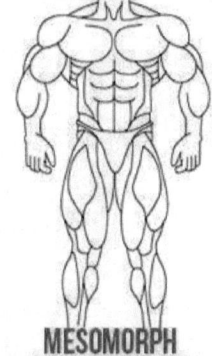
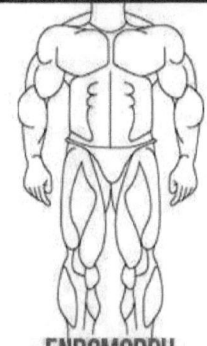

ECTOMORPH	MESOMORPH	ENDOMORPH
• TYPICALLY SKINNY	• ATHLETIC & RECTANGULAR SHAPE	• SOFT & ROUND BODY
• SMALL FRAME	• HARD BODY, DEFINED MUSCLES	• TYPICALLY "SHORT & STOCKY"
• LEAN MUSCLE MASS	• NATURALLY STRONG	• GAINS MUSCLE EASILY
• DOESN'T GAIN WEIGHT EASY	• GAINS MUSCLE EASILY	• GAINS FAT VERY EASILY
• FAST METABOLISM	• GAINS FAT EASIER THAN	• FINDS IT HARD TO LOSE FAT
• FLAT CHEST	ECTOMORPHS	• SLOW METABOLISM
• SMALL SHOULDERS	• BROAD SHOULDERS	• LARGE SHOULDERS

WORKOUT TYPE	WORKOUT TYPE	WORKOUT TYPE
SHORT & INTENSE, FOCUS ON BIG MUSCLE GROUPS EAT BEFORE BED TO PREVENT MUSCLE CATABOLISM	CARDIO & WEIGHT TRAINING RESPONDS BEST TO WEIGHT TRAINING WATCH CALORIE INTAKE	ALWAYS DO CARDIO TRAINING AND WEIGHT TRAINING WATCH CALORIE INTAKE

BUILD GREATER MUSCLE MASS THROUGH ACTIVE RECOVERY

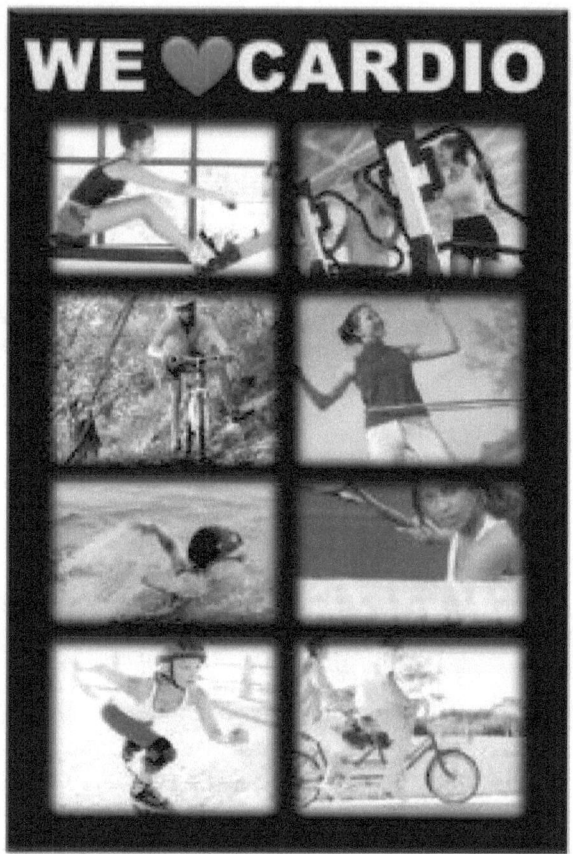

Rest has been mentioned throughout this text, but its importance cannot be overstated. Muscle mass derives from the microscopic tearing down and rebuilding of the tissues, and rebuilding occurs during periods of rest.

Active recovery (simply performing an easier activity) is important during a workout session.

- Muscles remain warmed up so that they can resume intense activity more quickly.

- The heart can move blood more efficiently – a sudden or prolonged decrease in activity causes blood to pool in the muscles since the heart is not pumping as fast.

- Staying active keeps you in the exercise frame of mind.

Active recovery is also important for people who feel they need to exercise daily. Along with splitting regular workouts up to focus on specific muscle groups on different days, engaging in completely different activities can provide a cardiovascular workout that works different muscles. Biking and swimming are two relatively low-impact options to offset strenuous strength exercises. Engaging in sports certainly incorporates functional movement and activities like yoga, hiking, Pilates, rock-wall climbing, and many others are fun as well as beneficial to overall fitness and strength.

Always pay attention to your body, and don't push past any warning signs. Feeling a little tired and sore is normal. Experiencing exhaustion or pain is an indication to rest and take the workout down a notch. Follow the basics of alternating days to work on specific muscle groups, or for extreme strength training, make sure to limit intense workouts to only 3 or 4 each week.

CONCLUSION

Anyone with the ability to move can increase their overall strength and fitness, lose weight, and improve their physical and emotional well-being. Starting with the simplest of steps, it is possible to create a calisthenics and bodyweight workout that will bring about these changes simply, for free and without having to go to a special facility. Just 20 to 30 minutes 3 to 4 days a week will create noticeable changes in just a few weeks.

Calisthenics and bodyweight training have been around since the time of the caveman and were the methods through which he was able grow, get strong, and live his life. These same functional movements can still provide excellent results today. Without weights, gadgets, or bulky equipment, anyone can increase muscle tone, strength, and mass and improve their range of motion and physical control. Just like the gladiators and ancient martial arts experts, men and women can develop plenty of strength, flexibility, and coordination by performing progressively more difficult variations of basic exercises.

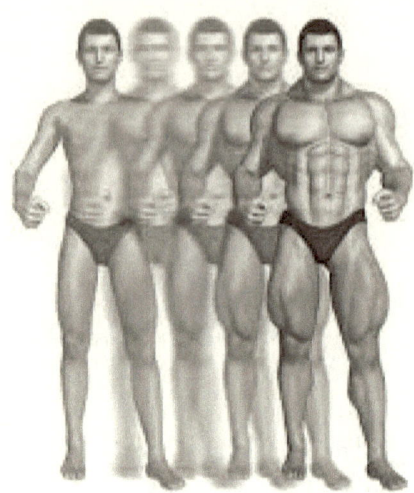

Understanding the basic process of how the body produces energy and the best types of food to ensure proper nutrition, anyone can maximize the effectiveness of a workout regimen. The key is to create a plan that incorporates not only better diet choices and increased physical activity but also adequate sleep and the reduction of stress. With the coordination of these factors, it is easy to achieve an improvement in overall health and well-being.

One of the most important factors in successful calisthenics and bodyweight workout programs is patience. The basics must be mastered before more difficult elements can be added, and the process just cannot be rushed. Not every individual will achieve the same results – that is simply not natural – but everyone can definitely improve their physical appearance and mental attitude with the proper attention to correct form and technique and following the right steps.

By reading this book and following the simple suggestions contained in it, you are on the way to leading a healthier, more active lifestyle with a body you are proud to show off. The first step is always the hardest so – put the book down and get moving!

ABOUT THE AUTHOR

John Powers was born into a low-income family in New York City. He knew from a young age that if he wanted to be able to go to a good college, he would need to find a way to get scholarships. He began examining a number of different skills, starting with art and ending with rugby. Though his school did not have their own rugby league, there was an intermural team in his area, which he joined at the age of twelve.

As one of the youngest and smallest kids on the team, he either had to sit out for most of the games or play positions that saw barely any action. He was never allowed in on the scrum. By the time he was fifteen, he was tired of sitting out and decided to see if there was something he could do to bulk up, become stronger and faster.

That's when John first encountered calisthenics. It wasn't just an umbrella term for all muscle building. It was a very narrow, very specific kind of weight lifting and muscle building that allowed him to get strong and fast in a very short amount of time.

Though he started researching and doing calisthenics just so he could improve his game, he also became interested in the exercise regimen as a theory, as a way for people to lose weight and bulk up at the same time. In lieu of a scholarship to a prestigious university, he joined the military, who paid for him, first to attend school, and then to return to the ranks to bulk up other soldiers.

Using what he had learned over the years and even developing his own techniques, he found that he could quickly improve the physical performance of his soldiers. His years of experience and his studies into the theories and mechanics of weight lifting and the body make him one of the country's foremost experts on calisthenics. It started as a way to make sure he saw more game time. It then became his passion, in university, on the field, and in his work.

Once he left the military, he opened his own personal training company, where he uses his skills to improve the bodies of all kinds of people. *Progressive Calisthenics* is a compilation of his workouts and nutrition advice, packaged just for you!

www.ingramcontent.com/pod-product-compliance
Lightning Source LLC
Chambersburg PA
CBHW020515290526
45786CB00002B/612